ACTIVE LIVING

The Miracle Medicine for a Long and Healthy Life

Gordon W. Stewart, MSc
3 S Group, Victoria, British Columbia

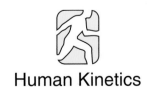

Human Kinetics

Library of Congress Cataloging-in-Publication Data

Stewart, Gordon W.
   Active living—The miracle medicine for a long
and healthy life / Gordon W. Stewart.
     p.   cm.
   Includes bibliographical references and index.
   ISBN 0-87322-678-X (pbk.)
   1. Exercise. 2. Physical fitness.   I. Title.
   RA781.S848   1995
   613.7'1--dc20   94-41353
                                CIP

ISBN: 0-87322-678-X

Developmental Editor: Rodd Whelpley; **Assistant Editors:** Julie Lancaster, Kirby Mittelmeier, and Jacqueline Blakley; **Copyeditor:** Molly Bentsen; **Proofreader:** Myla Smith; **Indexer:** Theresa J. Schaefer; **Typesetter:** Ruby Zimmerman; **Text Designer:** Stuart Cartwright; **Layout Artist:** Stuart Cartwright; **Cover Designer:** Stuart Cartwright; **Photographer (cover):** F-Stock; **Illustrator:** Keith Blomberg

Human Kinetics books are available at special discounts for bulk purchase. Special editions or book excerpts can also be created to specification. For details, contact the Special Sales Manager at Human Kinetics.

Printed in Hong Kong   10 9 8 7 6 5 4 3 2 1

Human Kinetics
P.O. Box 5076, Champaign, IL 61825-5076
1-800-747-4457

Canada: Human Kinetics, Box 24040, Windsor, ON N8Y 4Y9
1-800-465-7301 (in Canada only)

Europe: Human Kinetics, P.O. Box IW14, Leeds LS16 6TR, England
(44) 532 781708

Australia: Human Kinetics, 2 Ingrid Street, Clapham 5062, South Australia
(08) 371 3755

New Zealand: Human Kinetics, P.O. Box 105-231, Auckland 1
(09) 309 2259

This One's for Sandy

Writing is a solitary endeavor, and the most creative thoughts don't always come between 9 and 5. Over the years, my wife Sandy has allowed me the freedom and independence to pursue the writing life. But it's much more than this. Along the way, she has encouraged, supported, and contributed to projects I have done. Her experience as a teacher of physical education, biology, and dance lends an important perspective when she reviews things I have written. So does her sensible and balanced approach to life. She's my best critic and final "screen" before I let anything loose on the world. Her contributions to this book are subtle and many. For these, I'll always be grateful.

CONTENTS

INTRODUCTION
Setting the Record Straight

For years and years, fitness specialists have been encouraging people to set aside time for exercise. We've emphasized activities like running, cycling, and swimming to enhance cardiovascular endurance. Improve this component of fitness, we've always said, and better health will follow.

Well, there's good news for the great majority of people who have never responded to this message, for those who found it too much—too restricted, too time-consuming, too demanding. Too sweaty! Research now confirms that even modest levels of physical activity can have a positive effect on health. The route to health, we now know, can bypass huffing and puffing.

This isn't to suggest that we had it all wrong before. People who pursue vigorous activities stand to gain significant health benefits. Where we erred, perhaps, was in the scope of the message. In extolling the virtues of vigorous exercise, we may have given the impression that it was an all-or-nothing deal: that if you weren't prepared to get out there and "go for it," you might as well not bother at all.

Over the years, while the "exercise for fitness" approach dominated our thinking, scientists were working patiently to advance our understanding of the effects of physical activity on human health. The sum of their work now proves conclusively that even *moderate-intensity* activity has important pay-offs.

In the short term, regular, moderate, (*and*, of course, more demanding) activity can help you look better, feel better, and feel better about yourself. Over the long term, it can reduce your risk of coronary heart disease, improve your quality of life, and increase your life expectancy.

*H*ow Important Is Physical Activity?

The role of regular physical activity in preventing coronary heart disease is immense. The potential protection against heart disease that we would realize if everyone who is currently inactive became physically active would be greater than if all the people who smoke quit smoking.—Centers for Disease Control/Center for Health Promotion and Education

By embracing moderate-intensity activity, we broaden the spectrum of possibilities. Running, cycling, and swimming are still great. But so are dancing, hiking, working in the garden, and doing active chores around home.

Active living is the term being used as we take this broader approach, push beyond traditional fitness activities, and encourage people to find enjoyment in everyday things. On a very basic level, active living means including all sorts of simple activities in your daily routine, like walking to the corner store instead of taking the car, or climbing stairs instead of riding the elevator.

These are little things, but they all add up. We have learned the hard way that it's a grand leap from a life of inactivity to one that includes regular physical activity during your leisure time. We've learned this by witnessing all the people who have refused to take the leap, or who tried, and "failed," and then returned to their inactive ways.

Active living shortens the leap and turns it into a series of small, manageable steps. Individually they may not be much, and at first they may have no *measurable* effect on your health. But get into them and you may soon experience subtle, almost imperceptible, changes. Perhaps it'll be color in your cheeks, a spring in your stride, a little more energy, or some newfound enthusiasm.

Any one of these pleasant developments could encourage you to do more. Before you know it, you may be a lot more active than you used to be—and you will have accomplished this without even really trying.

Because this book is about *active living*, it's different from many of the other books that follow the narrower exercise-for-fitness approach. This book differs in three important ways:

- *It puts you in the driver's seat*. The exercise-for-fitness books tend to follow a cookbook, test-tube, do-this-and-you-get-that approach. *Active Living*, by contrast, takes a smorgasbord approach to physical activity. It presents a myriad of ideas to help you find activities that are right for you. Tastes and interests vary, and you must find your own appropriate medium for physical expression if habitual, lifelong activity is to result.

- *It goes beyond the physical*. Dr. Stanley Brown, a retired university physical education professor, once wisely observed that "most people will not exercise solely for the sake of their arteries." There are many important physical and practical benefits of active living, but there's more to it than this. Call it the spirit of movement, if you like. Few books advising people about physical activity even hint at this aspect. They take great care to show how *purposeful* activity is, without ever mentioning how *meaningful* it can be. Physical activity—active living—*is* a means to an end, but it is also a satisfying and rewarding end in itself.

- *It connects physical activity to other parts of life*. In the past, exercise has generally been presented as an add-on—something new, something else to do in your leisure time. While exercise may become a *part* of your life, active living is a *way of life*. As such, it recognizes that all things are related and affect one another. This is particularly true when we consider the health of our environment. Our activity choices are affected by *and* affect the world around us. Our individual actions all add up. They can make a difference—for better *or* for worse.

Activity for the '90s and Beyond

Running was at the forefront of the fitness boom in the 1970s. At times, it seemed as if every second person was training for the Boston Marathon. While many people were caught up in the enthusiasm, others were left in its wake.

The aerobics wave took over in the 1980s. Leotards and legwarmers were in, and going to a class was the thing to do. Fashions were important, and high-level fitness was prized above all.

These trends (and others) may have made physical activity seem less friendly and inviting than it really is. They may have served to exclude many people from an active way of life.

In the 1990s, we've settled down. *Active living* is helping us to regain a sense of balance. It values *all* kinds of activities and encourages choice—*your* choice.

Because active living is for everybody, this book caters to many needs and interests:

- *Inactive individuals* ("couch potatoes," if you like) will find the physical activity expectations realistic and the range of options palatable.

- *Modest movers* will be pleased to find that their current approach to physical activity is acceptable, will get some new ideas to broaden their repertoire, and should be encouraged to do a little more—to go beyond the basics.

- *Fitness enthusiasts* will find guidance to help them maintain a *sensible* approach to physical activity as well as motivation to try new things.

HERE'S WHAT'S HERE

There is an important difference between what is necessary and what is merely interesting. This is a book about *getting into* active living. There is so much to say about all the topics in this book. But for now, details can wait. I've tried hard to write about only what *needs* to be included.

If you look over the table of contents, you'll see that the chapter titles outline the essence of the active living message: *Get into active living. Make it part of your life.* Discover it has *something for every body,* and you may soon want to go *beyond the basics.* You'll be active *indoors* and *outdoors,* and you'll see how other healthy habits *complete the picture.*

To be more specific, following this introduction, chapters 1, 2, and 3 cover the many aspects of active living:

- *Chapter 1* explains what active living is all about, describes the benefits of an active lifestyle, and tells you how much activity you need to reap the rewards.

- *Chapter 2* gives you a chance to assess your current activity level, provides all kinds of ideas to help you fit physical activity into your day, and offers safety tips.

- *Chapter 3* advocates happy, active living for kids (with advice for parents, teachers, coaches, and others who care for and about them), and encourages activity for everyone, regardless of age or ability.

Chapters 4, 5, and 6 go beyond the basics, offering guidance and advice for a wide range of leisure-time activities:

- *Chapter 4* kicks off with six steps to success, important information no matter what you choose to do.

- *Chapter 5* covers indoor activities, with ideas for home exercise routines, suggestions for choosing a class or facility, and tips for court sports and team games.

- *Chapter 6* heads outdoors with a consumer guide and starter advice for walking and hiking, running, cycling, swimming, and a host of other activities.

Physical activity is only part of the picture, of course. Other habits also contribute to good health. To this end:

- *Chapter 7* offers practical tips for taking charge in the areas of diet and nutrition, stress management, smoking, and alcohol and other drugs. It concludes with a brief look at mental health and well-being.

Then it's back to active living.

- *Chapter 8* wraps things up and sets you on your way.

PLEASE DON'T READ THIS BOOK – USE *IT*

It's my hope that *Active Living* will become your friendly companion and guide, tattered and worn from use, not set on the shelf after a single reading.

Guidebooks are not necessarily designed for cover-to-cover reading. Focus on the information that is useful to you *now*. Why labor over advice on walking shoes if you're ready to head for the pool?

- *If you're quite inactive*, concentrate on chapters 1, 2, and 3. They provide what you need to get moving in a casual and comfortable way. Move on from there if you want to and when you're ready for it.

- *If you're active in your daily routine* but longing to do more in your leisure time, you can head for chapters 4, 5, and 6. (But do at least skim the first three chapters so you've got the gist of the active living message.)

- *If you feel you're not perfect(!)*, visit chapter 7. Many of us have health habits we'd like to refine. The modest changes suggested here can make a *big* difference to personal health.

Here are a few other suggestions:

- *Chart your course.* The table of contents lists the topics included in each chapter. The introduction to each chapter elaborates on what's covered there. The index at the back of the book helps you find specific information. Use these guides to good advantage—to help you get the most out of the book.

- *Keep a pencil handy.* You'll find a variety of self-quizzes, checklists, and forms throughout the book. Chapter 4, for example, includes *PAR-Q*—a preactivity questionnaire for those who plan to become much more physically active. You may have the urge to skip past these elements and keep on reading. Resist it! If you use these tools properly, the information in the book will be more *personally* meaningful. This in turn will help you be more successful in whatever you choose to do.

- *Seek additional advice.* For some people, this book should not be their sole guide. A number of health concerns are covered in chapter 3. If any of them affects you, discuss your physical activity plans with your doctor or another health professional. If you are interested in a fitness appraisal and personal advice, see pages 123-124. Use this information to help you find someone with the qualifications and experience to guide you properly. Finally, to assist you as your interest grows, a short and select reading list is provided on pages 125-127.

- *Get to the end.* No matter how you plan to read and use the book, please read chapter 8. It covers an important part of the active living theme.

One final suggestion: Be patient. Don't rush or force things no matter what activities you pursue. Push too hard and the body rebels. Treat it sensibly and with respect and it will perform remarkably.

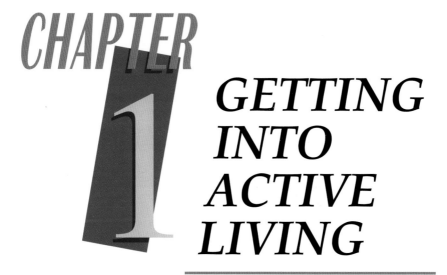

CHAPTER 1

GETTING INTO ACTIVE LIVING

*T*his chapter builds a foundation for the information that follows it. It includes three sections:

• ***UNDERSTANDING IT*** explains just what active living is about. It's not all that complicated, but active living *is* more than simply living actively.

• ***REAPING THE REWARDS*** outlines the merits of an active lifestyle. There are many good reasons to be a "modest mover."

• ***GETTING ENOUGH*** charts the new route to health, outlining the amount of activity you need to attain the benefits discussed. This section also defines a few terms—exercise, fitness, health, wellness, etc.—to help you keep things straight.

Time now to set out en route to active living.

UNDERSTANDING IT

 *verything has been thought of before.
The problem is to think of it again.*

—Goethe

Active living is not a revolutionary idea—it's evolutionary. It has its roots in the past while showing the way to the future. It's a return to the basics—to simplicity, to moderation, to variety. It recognizes the joys, and values, and benefits of many kinds of activities. It means pursuing activities you find useful, pleasurable, and satisfying.

Active living is about *healthy* choices—*your* choices. The physical activities you do will depend on many things. They may be different when you're sixty years old than when you're thirty. Different for students than for busy parents. Different depending on your abilities and your interests. And different as a result of family traditions and cultural heritage.

Active living is clearly different things to different people, but it has something for everyone.

ACTIVE LIVING AND THE INDIVIDUAL

Active living means taking things in stride—doing what comes naturally. It's gardening and golfing, dancing and dodgeball. It's squash and swimming, walking and wheeling. It's playing in the park with the kids, even washing the car or mowing the lawn!

It's as simple as this and more than this. Active living is

- finding a balance, a comfortable combination of activities you can enjoy, not rush to fit in;
- being active alone (to unwind) if you need it;
- using active time with others to share experiences;
- cooperating in a group activity or competing in a game;
- trying new activities—learning and self-discovery;

- slowing down and enjoying the simple pleasure of being in motion;
- experiencing the outdoors—its changing seasons; its birds, and trees, and sunsets; its morning fogs and evening breezes.

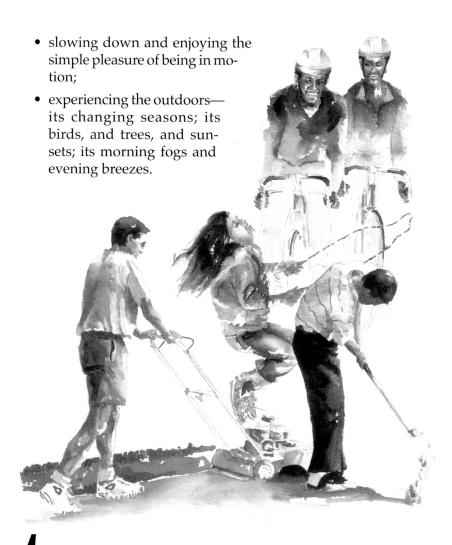

A ctive living is a way of life in which physical activity is valued and integrated into daily life.

ACTIVE LIVING AND COMMUNITY

Active living goes beyond the individual. It involves cooperation and caring, peace and harmony.

It means creating communities that are friendly and supportive—that make it easy for active living to be a way of life. This includes "communities" in all their forms—apartment blocks, neighborhoods, workplaces, schools, and so on.

In this regard, active living involves

- reaching out and helping others in their efforts to be active;

- helping to make your own communities healthier, safer, cleaner—in short, more livable.

Active living also encompasses the idea of living lightly on the land, as the advocates for a healthy environment so wisely advise.

In the end, active living is enjoying life one step at a time.

- First you *choose* it. This involves understanding the full meaning of active living and being aware of your alternatives, then creating opportunities.

- Next you *value* it. You become comfortable with your choice, supporting family and friends who share your enthusiasm but accepting others who don't.

- Finally, you *act*. You follow through on your choice and experience the pleasures of physical activity. You live a life that's right for you, in tune with others, and in harmony with the world around you.

REAPING THE REWARDS

 f you could bottle everything you get from physical activity and sell it at the pharmacy, it would go for a hefty price.

—Dr. George Sheehan

Exercise specialists have long touted the importance of regular activity, but the topic has finally made the big time. With the mounting evidence from their careful research done over the years, *physical inactivity* is now officially recognized as a *risk factor* (in and of itself) for cardiovascular disease. It joins three other biggies on the list: smoking, high blood pressure, and high blood cholesterol.

This risk factor designation has been bestowed by a number of important organizations: the International Federation and Society for Cardiology, the World Health Organization, the American Heart Association, and the Heart and Stroke Foundation of Canada.

There are *many* benefits to being a modest mover—an "active liver." But you cannot "store up" these benefits; you can only continue to experience them as long as you keep up the physical-activity habit. Some benefits are subtle and long term; others are for the here and now. Every one of them is supported by scientific research.

LONG-TERM BENEFITS

Long-term benefits deal mainly with heart health and avoiding problems. Physical activity becomes a kind of "preventive medicine." Some benefits help prevent disability and loss of independence, and they certainly become more important as we get older.

Get a pencil and, as you read through this first list, check (✓) the benefits that are meaningful to you.

LONG-TERM BENEFITS OF ACTIVE LIVING

Regular physical activity is important to me because . . .

☐ it strengthens the heart and lungs and improves circulation.

☐ it helps control blood pressure.

☐ it can help to reduce blood fat and cholesterol.

☐ it may boost the body's ability to ward off colds and other illnesses.

☐ it helps to maintain balance, coordination, and agility.

☐ it keeps the muscles supple and strong and the joints mobile.

☐ it strengthens the bones, offering some protection against osteoporosis.

HERE AND NOW

The benefits in the next list are about *today*. They are things you can achieve, enjoy, or experience almost immediately. Take your pencil again, and check (✓) any of the items that apply.

EVERYDAY BENEFITS OF ACTIVE LIVING

I would like to . . .

- ☐ look better.
- ☐ have more energy and stamina.
- ☐ get more fun out of life.
- ☐ cope better with daily stresses.
- ☐ relax more and sleep more soundly.
- ☐ enjoy my food more and be less preoccupied with my weight.
- ☐ have a greater sense of control over my life.
- ☐ feel better about myself.

How did you do? There is no passing grade, no magic number of checkmarks you should have on these two health-benefit lists. But the more you have, the better, and the more inclined you will be to embrace active living and make it a way of life.

Many people choose to become more active for the reasons on the long-term benefits list—because it's good for them, because they know they should. But few people stay with activity for these reasons alone.

No, you have to *feel better*, too. And that's what the everyday benefits list is all about. Ask people a few weeks into a new activity routine what they think it's doing for them, and somewhere in their testimonials you almost always hear the simple but important phrase "I feel better."

This "feeling better" comes in many guises. A forty-year-old father of two young boys says, "I can now throw the ball and chase my sons around without getting tired." Another person says she finds an improvement in her golf swing and more enjoyment in her game due to her exercise routine.

A most heartfelt description of feeling better came from a participant in an activity program I used to run, when she responded to a questionnaire asking what value she found in the class.

Her response, which is reproduced here, is a wonderful account of how active living rewards you twice. It rewards you immediately in the pleasure of the moment. And it rewards you over time through improved health, well-being, and quality of life.

WHAT VALUE DID YOU FIND IN YOGAEROBICS*?

It is significant. I arrive a lazy, tired, and rheumatically cranky middle-aged lady, and I leave full of vitality and well-being toward the world in general. I have not felt so happy for a long time. This overflows into my working life, where—I do not need to detail—one encounters so many irritants. Of course, I still succumb to them. . . . But I find I am better able to cope. I sincerely mean this.

I am less winded.

I think I look better, and to one who has reached face-lift time, this is important.

There is the satisfaction of seeing neglected limbs becoming . . . very, very gradually in my case . . . supple.

I consider Yogaerobics ideal for me. It is interesting to observe that even after walking/running almost a mile, one's limbs are very much out of condition when used for a different type of movement. Also, one complements the active approach with the contemplative.

Finally, one has the opportunity to observe the insidious result of not using one's body effectively over the years.

*A yoga and easy walking/running class

GETTING ENOUGH

 ny activity is better than no activity from a
health perspective.

—Dr. Steven Blair

Active living is definitely on the move. This casual, low-key approach to physical activity is an easy pill to swallow. And it offers many benefits, as the previous section explained.
But the big question is this: How much is enough?
The answer is, a lot less than we used to think.

THE NEW ROUTE TO HEALTH

In the past we have tended to focus on *exercise* to improve *physical fitness*. We encouraged people to pursue vigorous aerobic activities (running, cycling, swimming) for the sake of their cardiovas-

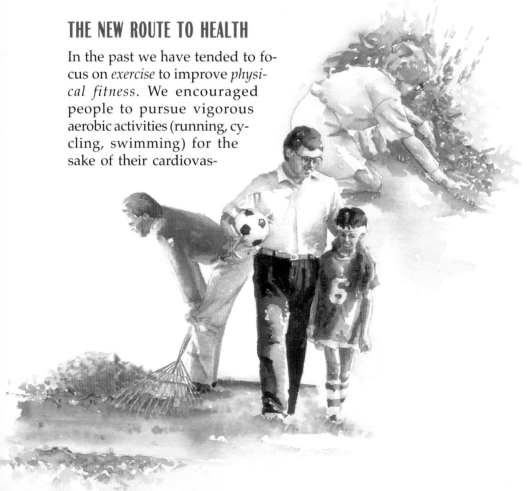

cular endurance, or stamina. This in turn would lead to better health.

But as the body of research grows, it's increasingly clear that more modest levels of *physical activity* can have a positive effect on *health*. A quick look at the Heart Rate Target Zone chart on page 48 helps to demonstrate this broader view.

If the focus is on improving cardiovascular endurance, scientists agree that we should exercise at a level between 70% and 85% of our predicted maximum heart rate. This is shown by the area shaded yellow in the chart. But we now know that *health* benefits accrue at lower levels of exertion. This addition to the Heart Rate Target Zone is shown by the green band in the chart, with 55% of predicted maximum heart rate as the threshold (or lower) level. Anything that increases the heart rate to this minimum level is considered *moderate-intensity* activity. For most people, the everyday active living ideas noted earlier—brisk walking, gardening, raking leaves, and the like—are demanding enough to do the trick.

In support of modest moving, *Public Health Reports* offers the following summary:

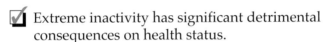 Extreme inactivity has significant detrimental consequences on health status.

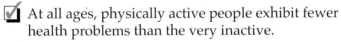 At all ages, physically active people exhibit fewer health problems than the very inactive.

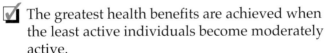 The greatest health benefits are achieved when the least active individuals become moderately active.

A large number of scientific studies done over several decades have brought us to this level of understanding.

Early studies on coronary heart disease (CHD) and physical activity focused on *occupational activity*. The most famous of these involved double-decker bus drivers and conductors in London, England, and longshoremen in San Francisco, California. In both cases, the more active individuals—bus conductors and cargo handlers—had significantly less CHD than did their less active fellow workers.

Similar results have been found when looking at leisure-time physical activities. Large-scale studies of heart health done in Massachusetts, Hawaii, and Finland, for example, all demonstrated lower coronary heart disease risk in those who were more physically active during their leisure time.

Other important research confirms that moderate-intensity activity pays off.* For example:

- One study, conducted at the Institute for Aerobics Research in Dallas, Texas, followed more than 13,000 women and men over eight years. The death rates from all causes for those with moderate levels of fitness were significantly less than for those with low fitness levels. A brisk walk of as little as thirty minutes a day is sufficient to provide the modest level of fitness that seems to offer protection from CHD.

- The *Multiple Risk Factor Intervention Trial* (or Mr. Fit), conducted by the University of Minnesota had similar results. A seven-year follow-up of more than 12,000 middle-aged men showed that those involved in moderate leisure-time physical activity experienced about a third less fatal coronary heart diseases than those in the low-activity group. Moderate activities that fill the bill include gardening, yard work, home repairs, dancing, swimming, and home exercise.

- A third study, done at Stanford University's School of Medicine, showed significant fitness improvement in people who did thirty minutes of moderate-intensity activity daily for eight weeks. Improvement came *regardless* of whether the activity was continuous or done in three bouts of ten minutes each.

This final study helps to demonstrate that total energy expended throughout the day—not one continuous activity session—is what's important. Bouts of activity as brief as five minutes seem to produce the much desired health benefits. Fitting activity into your day in this manner is part of what active living is all about. Short walks, taking the stairs, and the like, *do* add up.

---

*For more on the research which supports the health benefits of physical activity, see the Research Reports portion of the *Suggested Reading* list at the back of this book.

*E*nough's Enough

Modest health benefits can come from adding as little as 500 calories of energy expenditure a week to a *very* inactive lifestyle. But the benefits really begin to click in at 1,000 calories a week of moderate-intensity activity, and they increase as you move up to 2,000 calories and more. If you're inactive now, take it one step at a time. Aim for the 1,000-calorie mark for starters, and consider 2,000 calories a nice goal to strive for over the long term.

To give some practical examples, *any one* of the following will burn about 1,000 calories:

- 5 hours of housework
- 3-1/2 hours of gardening or yard work
- 3 hours of walking
- 2-1/2 hours of ice-skating
- 2 hours of downhill skiing
- 2 hours of tennis
- 1-3/4 hours of racquetball or squash
- 1-1/2 hours of running (at 10 minutes/mile)

It's common, of course, to mix and match. Your 1,000 calories for the week could be nine holes of golf (no cart!), some yard work, and two or three walks to the store. Or it could be a couple of sessions of tennis. The choice *is* yours!

*E*nough's Enough takes a calorie-counting approach to active living. Putting it another way, the American College of Sports Medicine says, "Every adult should *accumulate* 30 minutes or more of moderate-intensity activity over the course of *most days* of the week."

KEEPING THE WORDS STRAIGHT

I've tossed around a few words here in explaining how much activity is enough. It might be good to define these terms before moving on. I do it to help keep things straight, but I worry nonetheless. If there's a chance you'll yawn and nod off while reading this book, this could be where it happens. Stay with me!

For the record:

- *Physical activity* is any body movement produced by skeletal muscles and resulting in energy expenditure. It can be categorized into occupational, household, leisure-time, and other activities.

- *Exercise*, a subset of physical activity, is planned, structured, and repetitive. Its main objective is to improve or maintain physical fitness.

- *Physical fitness* comprises a set of attributes that are either health related or skill (or performance) related. *Health-related fitness* includes cardiovascular endurance (stamina), muscular strength and endurance, flexibility, and body composition (more on this in chapter 5). *Skill/performance-related fitness* covers such elements as balance, speed, and agility.

Along with these components, *physical fitness* has been defined as the ability to carry out daily tasks with vigor and alertness, without undue fatigue, and with ample energy to enjoy leisure-time pursuits and to meet unforeseen emergencies.

Continuing with this building-block approach, physical fitness is one aspect of health. *Health* has physical, social, and psychological dimensions, each characterized on a continuum with positive and negative poles. Positive health is associated with a capacity to enjoy life and to withstand challenges; it is not merely the absence of disease. Health has also been nicely described as a "resource for everyday life."

What about wellness? *Wellness* is a holistic concept, describing a state of positive health in the individual and comprising physical, social, and psychological well-being.

There are those who say wellness is something new, something different from, or broader than, health. I don't buy that for a minute. The definitions of health and wellness have more similarities than differences. They're only words. Get to discussing them and you're soon doing the semantics shuffle.

Personally, I like the word *health*—always have, always will. Others hang their hats on wellness. You can call it what you like.

As for *active living*, it was defined at length in the first section of this chapter. Physical activity *is* a big part of it, but there are social and psychological aspects, too, just as there are for health. So you really can get there from here.

THE FEELING-BETTER BAROMETER

The studies I discussed earlier tend to focus on the long-term benefits of moderate-intensity physical activity (as outlined on p. 5). The emphasis is very much on disease prevention and increased life expectancy.

But how you feel today is obviously important, too. That's where the everyday benefits of active living (covered on p. 6) come in. These tend to be less tangible, more individual, more personal. They're harder to put a finger on, harder to quantify, but they're important in their own right.

Everyone has his or her own feeling-better barometer. The forty-year-old father, the golfer, and the Yogaerobics participant mentioned earlier are testament to this. You'll soon discover what active living has in store for you.

CHAPTER 2
MAKING ACTIVE LIVING PART OF YOUR LIFE

*T*hrough ingenuity and inventions, we have managed to *take out* much of the physical activity we used to get from our daily routines. Clothes washers and dryers, automatic dishwashers, and electronic remotes spare us physical effort. So do garage door openers, snowblowers, elevators and escalators, and other modern conveniences. They're little things, but they add up.

This chapter is about *putting* physical activity *back* into your routine. It's about doing a little more, a little bit at a time. It's about moving more, and moving more often.

There are three sections:

• *TAKING STOCK* calls for some thoughtful *in*action. It's a chance to confirm what's important to you, assess how you're doing now, and determine what changes you might make.

• *DOING YOUR BEST EVERY DAY* offers a smorgasbord of ideas to help you *activate* your daily routine—to act in ways that are good for you and good for the environment.

• *TAKING CARE* covers some general safety and injury prevention issues. It's advice for enjoyable, trouble-free activity—whatever you choose to do.

TAKING STOCK

When there are choices to consider and decisions to make, some simple planning helps. If you feel you should be more active during your *normal daily routine*, spend a few minutes completing the *Basic Action Plan*. Look over the active living ideas in the next section if it will help trigger your thinking. Once you've completed your plan, you can put it into action!

BASIC ACTION PLAN

When it comes to active living during my daily routine, how am I doing now?

What changes would I like to make? What else would I like to do?

What would help me do it?

Here is how I ought to get started:

The *Advanced Action Plan* will help if you would like to be more active in your *leisure time*. The questions get at your motives, interests, and aptitudes relating to physical activity. They're like pieces of a puzzle that, properly constructed, will help you choose activities that are just right for you. Use your responses in the advanced plan along with the tips and advice in chapter 4 when you want to go beyond the basics. (Use a separate sheet of paper if you need more space.)

ADVANCED ACTION PLAN

What did I like most (and least) about being active when I was younger?

What physical activities did I really enjoy when I was younger?

What are my main reasons for wanting to be more active now?

What activities have I always wanted to try but never really had the opportunity to do?

What other activities seem interesting now and would be worth exploring?

What are my major obstacles to being more active? How can I overcome them?

Important goals of my program are these:

Considering all of these things, here are the activities that make the most sense for me now:

DOING YOUR BEST EVERY DAY

When it comes to active living, no change you might make is too little or unimportant. Numerous small changes can make a *big* difference—for you *and* for the environment.

FITTING PHYSICAL ACTIVITY INTO YOUR DAY

The following lists are by no means complete. They're included to give you some general ideas for being more active during your normal daily routine: at home, at school, at work, and at play. You'll surely think of other things you can do. (There are spaces at the bottom of each list where you can add your own ideas.)

If you completed the *Basic Action Plan*, start with one or two of the activities you recorded there. Whatever activities you choose, they should be easy and right for you now. Give them a try for a while. Make them part of your routine. Once they become habit, choose a couple more and start the process again. If you like, check (✓) activities as you choose them—*and do them!*—to help you keep track of your efforts.

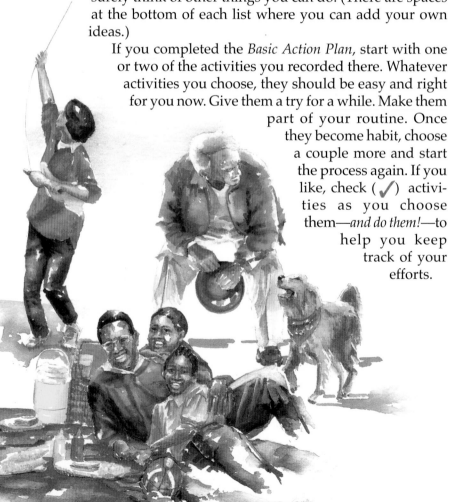

ACTIVE LIVING . . .

. . . AT HOME

Put gusto into *all* your indoor and outdoor chores around the house:

❏ Devise a simple bending and stretching routine. Do it while you brush your teeth, watch TV, or wait for water to boil.

❏ Dust, vacuum, and wash windows regularly.

❏ Make your own bread.

❏ Create a flower garden, or use planters on your porch or balcony.

❏ Tend a garden plot and grow some of your own vegetables.

❏ Do active outdoor work. Dig weeds, rake leaves, chop wood, push a wheelbarrow.

❏ Use a push mower to cut the grass.

❏ Wash the car. Give it a good shine!

❏ Sweep the driveway; clean out the garage.

❏ Shovel—don't blow!—the snow.

❏ _____

❏ _____

. . . AT SCHOOL

Develop good habits at school:

❏ Take physical education or other activity classes every chance you get.

❏ Be active during breaks between classes.

❏ Jump rope. Ride a skateboard.

(continued)

❏ Join clubs that involve physical activity—hiking, dance, or another choice.

❏ Participate in intramurals. Try all sorts of new games and sports.

❏ Sign up for school teams.

❏ _____

❏ _____

... AT WORK

Set a good example, and push for active living in the workplace:

❏ Take the stairs instead of the elevator.

❏ Go for a lunchtime stroll.

❏ Take short stretch breaks when you need them.

❏ Plan a formal stretch break program for your colleagues.

❏ Search out unused space and turn it into a group activity area.

❏ Use nearby parks and facilities for employee activity programs.

❏ Organize recreational activities—teams, leagues, clubs, and the like.

❏ Push for on-site showers and change rooms for activity participants.

❏ Lobby for covered, secure bicycle parking so employees can cycle to work.

❏ _____

❏ _____

... AT PLAY

Take the child in you out to play:

- ☐ Go for a stroll. Feed the ducks.
- ☐ Take a hike. Have a picnic. Laugh a lot.
- ☐ Throw a Frisbee. Fly a kite. Swing a hockey stick.
- ☐ Go bird-watching, or stargazing.
- ☐ Dance vigorously—and often.
- ☐ Include all kinds of active hobbies in your leisure time.
- ☐ Use vacations to try out new activities, then add them to your routine when you get home.
- ☐ _____
- ☐ _____

... EN ROUTE

When going from place to place, make the *active* choice:

- ☐ Walk, skate, cycle or wheel on short trips and outings—to the mailbox, the store, the park.
- ☐ Commute by bicycle part or all of the way to work or school.
- ☐ Take public transportation and walk whenever possible—to work, on errands, around town.
- ☐ _____
- ☐ _____

*T*ime to Play

Millions of kids *can't* be wrong—playing *is* fun! And it isn't just for the young. Introducing active play into our lives will help counter the stresses of adult life. Simple play is just fine. You don't need fancy equipment or special clothing. Playing is doing, *not* having.

GOING GREEN

Walking woodland trails, picnicking, bird-watching, beachcombing, and swimming are all enjoyable outdoor pursuits. But for these and many other activities, a clean and healthy environment is important to the experience. The physical activities we choose in turn affect the environment.

Active living recognizes this relationship. It encourages activities that allow you to appreciate and enjoy but at the same time respect the natural environment.

"Active commuting"—walking, running, or cycling to and from work or school—may be the most obvious and visible example of this. By making the *active* choice whenever we can, we reap personal health benefits while treating the environment in a caring manner.

Never has the "going green" philosophy been more on our minds—*or* more important. Beyond active commuting, there are many simple things we all can do to protect the world around us.

Reduce, reuse, and recycle is not only a catch phrase for the environmental movement but by now a way of life for many, many people. Those at the forefront of the movement suggest other *R*s we should add to the list—*refuse, rehabilitate, restore, rethink* and *reform* are among them.

Many of the active living ideas listed earlier in the chapter cover the *R* words. They involve making the *right* choice. Here are some reminders, along with a few related suggestions:

- Prepare a garden plot, and grow your own vegetables. To complete the cycle, compost your yard waste and return the organic richness to the soil.

- Choose foods as close to their natural state as possible. Avoid excessive packaging in foods or anything you buy. (Here's the *refuse* part of the *R*-word family in action. Our collective actions *can* lead to change.)

- Don't cut down a tree unless it's absolutely necessary. Plant a new one every chance you get.

- Rest the car, not your body. Be an active commuter whenever you can.

- Choose human-powered leisure-time activities. Leave the powerboat at the dock, the snowmobile in the garage.

- Adopt a favorite natural place—a local park, a trail, a stream. Get a group together and commit yourselves to keeping your place safe and clean. Every "litter bit" helps!

- Lobby for change in your community. Push for projects that *care for* and *clean up* the environment. Turn successful projects into an ongoing, regular way of life.

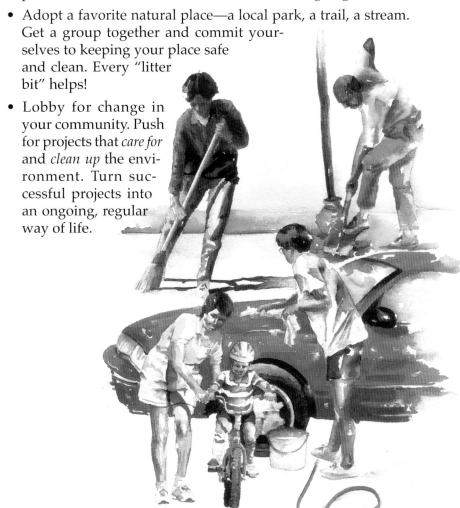

By doing these sorts of things we stay in touch with nature. Perhaps then we can truly know and understand the words attributed to Chief Seattle: "The earth does not belong to man; man belongs to the earth. This we know. All things are connected like the blood which unites one family. All things are connected."

TAKING CARE

The fastest way to *in*active living is to suffer an injury, have an accident, or experience some kind of mishap or setback.

An important first step to trouble-free activity is to look after your back and your knees. Tips to this end are included here, followed by some advice for safe activity in the heat (and sun) and the cold.

BACK AND KNEE BASICS

Back pain is a tangible problem. If you've got it, you know it! Fortunately, *most* back pain is preventable, or easily rectified if you already have it. What it takes is a little effort and care. Here are some tips to help:

- *Keep fit.* Active living can help you maintain a good general level of physical fitness. This in turn will contribute to "back fitness."

- *Stretch and strengthen.* Strong and supple muscles in the trunk, low back, and legs are particularly important. (See *Stretch It* and *Strength Fit* in chapter 5 for easy every-other-day routines.)

- *Reduce excess weight.* Extra weight in the abdominal area can cause an excessive forward tilt of the spine and put pressure on the lower back. (See *Eating Right* in chapter 7 for some tips and advice.)

- *Pay attention to posture.* Proper posture involves correct positioning of all levels of the spine. Keep your head over your shoulders—don't poke your chin forward. Keep your shoulders level, slightly back, and relaxed. If you have an excessive forward curve in your lower back, reduce it by gently tucking in your stomach, tightening your buttocks, and bending your knees slightly.

- *Practice good posture every day.* Use these elements of good posture in all your daily activities—sitting, standing, and walking.

Set up your work areas (in the kitchen, at the office, etc.) so they are easy on your back. Wear comfortable shoes with low heels.

- *Lift with care.* Stand close to the object you plan to lift, with feet comfortably apart to give a stable base. Lift with your legs— don't make your back do all the work. Keep the object close to your body. Lift slowly and smoothly, and avoid twisting.

Although much attention these days seems to focus on the back, you mustn't forget the knees. Here are some tips for protecting them:

- *Stoop to it.* Gardening and other chores and activities around home may require a lot of bending, stooping, and kneeling. Pace yourself during these activities, and don't overdo it.

- *Get good shoes.* Running, aerobics, court games, and other activities place specific demands on the body. Whatever you do, wear shoes that provide adequate support for your feet. The cushioning that good shoes offer will help protect your legs from injury.

- *Keep your legs strong.* If the muscles that stabilize the knee joint are strong and supple, they help to "cushion" movement, reduce stress on the knees, and prevent injuries. The "Strength Fit" routine on pages 70-75 provides some exercises to help here.

Discomfort and injuries *can* be avoided. If you treat your back and your knees sensibly, they shouldn't give you any trouble.

IN THE HEAT (AND SUN)

Activity in warm weather requires special care and attention. Whether it's gardening, tennis, a walk, or some other pleasurable endeavor, here are guidelines to consider:

- *Dress for the weather.* Wear comfortable clothing to suit the weather *and* your activity. Go for light colors on sunny days.

- *Protect yourself from the sun.* Minimize your exposure during the hottest part of the day (10:00 a.m. to 3:00 p.m.). Use waterproof sunscreen with a sun protection factor (SPF) of 15 or higher; look for one that protects against both ultraviolet (UV) A and B radiation. Reapply it regularly as required if you're perspiring or swimming. Wear a wide-brimmed hat and sunglasses offering UV protection.

- *Don't overdo it.* Do less (and less intense) activity than you would on cooler days. Take rest breaks when you need them.

- *Drink lots of water.* To avoid dehydration, drink plenty of water before, during, and after physical activity. (A couple of big mouthfuls every 15 minutes or so will do the trick.) When you're done, drink a cup of water for every half pound of weight lost during your session.

Overexertion in hot weather should be avoided as it can lead to heat exhaustion or, in the extreme, heatstroke.

Signs of heat exhaustion include pale skin, profuse sweating, and a weak, rapid pulse. To treat it, stop activity, lie down in a cool (shady) spot, and drink cool water. Increased water intake over the next few days is also recommended.

Early signs of heatstroke are hot and dry skin and a strong, rapid pulse. Other signs are headache, muscle cramps, dizziness and blurred vision, and incoherent speech. The victim may even lose consciousness. This is a serious condition requiring rapid cooling and immediate medical attention.

OUT IN THE COLD

Activity in cold weather can be safe and enjoyable if you take proper precautions. Whether you're shoveling snow, playing hockey, or heading off to ski, here are some things to remember:

- *Dress for the weather.* Layers of loose-fitting clothing trap air and provide good insulation. The inner layer should be absorbent and help "wick" perspiration away from the skin. The middle layer (or layers) should provide warmth. The outer layer should be water repellent and wind resistant. (Layers also let you remove or add clothing to adjust to your activity level, wind conditions, etc.) Finally, use sunscreen and sunglasses on bright days. (See the advice in the previous section.)

- *Top things off.* Keep your hands, feet, and head warm. Wear mittens or gloves, warm socks, a stocking cap, and even a face mask on particularly cold days.

- *Beware of the wind.* Take the windchill factor into account, and dress accordingly. As much as possible, plan walking, hiking, and skiing routes so the wind is at your back near the end of your session.

- *Watch for fatigue.* Don't push yourself in extremely cold weather. And always drink plenty of water, even if you don't feel thirsty. Water is important when you're active, regardless of the weather.
- *Use the buddy system.* If you're off the beaten track—hiking or cross-country skiing, for example—try to be active with a companion. Keep your eye on one another, and watch for warning signs of exposure to the cold.
- *Don't dawdle.* When your activity is finished, get inside and change into dry clothing as soon as possible.

Of the problems that can result from exposure to the cold, frostbite and hypothermia are the most serious.

Frostbite occurs when so much heat is lost that the water in tissue close to the skin freezes. The ears, face, fingers, and toes are most susceptible. Early signs include skin that is waxy, white, numb, tingly, and cold.

Hypothermia is a potentially fatal condition in which the core body temperature falls dangerously below normal. The earliest signs include numbness in the hands and feet and slight shivering. Continued exposure can lead to more intense shivering, slurred speech, drowsiness, even a feeling of exhaustion.

When any of these symptoms appears, it is crucial to seek shelter, get into dry clothing, and have a snack (preferably a hot drink). Serious cases require immediate medical attention.

dministering First Aid

Everyone should have the ability to respond to injuries and accidents when they occur. This requires adequate knowledge and the right tools. Training in first aid and CPR is essential. Armed with this information—and a good first-aid kit—you'll be able to *take care* during physical activity. Here is a list of essential supplies. Your particular setting and activities may warrant additional items.

Adhesive (athletic) tape (3.8 cm)	2 rolls
Antibiotic ointment	1 tube
Bandages (strip/finger/knuckle)	20
Cotton-tipped applicators	10
Elastic bandage, 7.5 cm	1
Elastic bandage, 10 or 15 cm	1
Gauze pads (sterile)	10
Gloves (latex)	2 pairs
Plastic bags (for ice)	4
Pocket mask for cardiopulmonary resuscitation	1
Prepackaged cloth wipes	6
Saline or antiseptic solution	1 bottle
Scissors	1 pair
Safety pins	6
Skin lubricant (e.g., petroleum jelly) (3-oz jar)	1
Sterile needles (5/8", 25 gauge)	5
Sterile wound closures	5 packages
Sterile nonadherent pads	10
Tape adherent (4-oz can)	1
Tongue depressors	2
Towel	1
Triangular bandages	2

Pen, notepad, emergency telephone numbers, coins for the telephone, and a current first-aid manual.

Let's hope that once your kit is ready, chances are you'll rarely have to use it. (This is based on the same theory that says when you've got an umbrella it's less likely to rain.)

CHAPTER

3

SOMETHING FOR EVERY BODY

*T*he main point of this chapter is that active living is *inclusive*. It's for everyone, regardless of age, ability, or other personal circumstances.

Two sections offer special information and advice:

• *GETTING STARTED EARLY* pushes the point that active living begins at home. It includes a variety of suggestions for happy, active-living kids at home, at school, *and* at play.

• *SUITING YOURSELF* is for individuals who might need a bit of extra advice. It discusses common health concerns that will affect active living choices. It also considers aging and activity and other challenges. Tips and advice are included throughout.

Active living *is* good for the body—*every* body!

GETTING STARTED EARLY

When it comes to kids and physical activity, things aren't what they used to be. Children and youth today are less active and less fit than in earlier generations. There are all sorts of reasons for this, television and video games among them. While these developments are worrisome, we *can* turn them around.

Good active living habits should be developed at an early age. They start at home and are then nurtured and reinforced at school and through sports, games, and other organized activities.

ACTIVE LIVING BEGINS AT HOME

Parents who want their children to be active should follow three cardinal rules:

- Set a good example.
- Play together whenever you can.
- Encourage and support children's participation in all kinds of physical activities.

Research on children and physical activity shows the crucial role that parents play. *More active* parents have more active preschoolers, more active preadolescents, and more active adolescents.

It all starts at the beginning. Infants should be encouraged to move whenever possible. All that arm swinging and leg kicking is great. (Call it "midget aerobics" if you like!)

In toddlers, the transition from crawling to standing and walking is a natural and normal part of growing and experiencing movement.

Preschoolers explore a broader range of movement as they learn to run, jump, climb, and throw. Informal and friendly play will do much to nurture their love of physical activity.

School-age children enjoy the challenge of more formal games and activities. Basic coordination is well developed by about age seven. At age eight, children are playing more games than at any other time. We should take advantage of this—parents (and grandparents!) can help.

My friend Bill Ross, a retired university professor and growth and development specialist, says that older generations know more

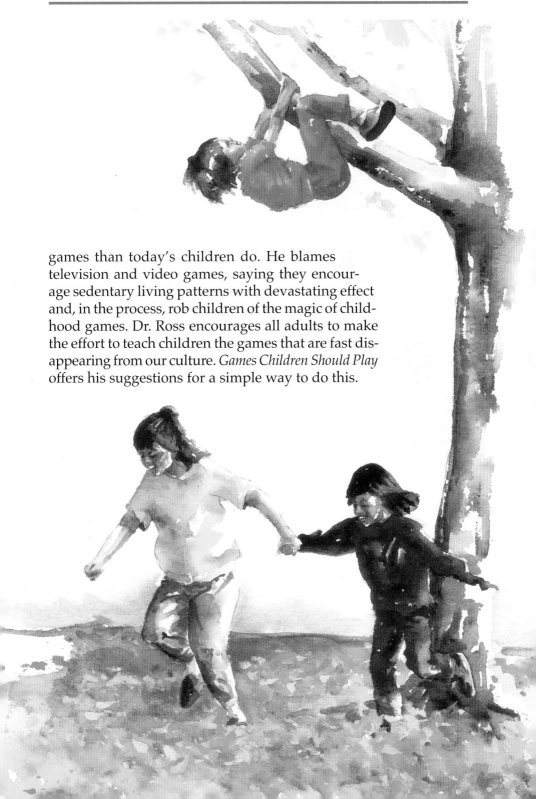

games than today's children do. He blames television and video games, saying they encourage sedentary living patterns with devastating effect and, in the process, rob children of the magic of childhood games. Dr. Ross encourages all adults to make the effort to teach children the games that are fast disappearing from our culture. *Games Children Should Play* offers his suggestions for a simple way to do this.

ames Children Should Play

To teach children the fun games of your youth, keep these guidelines in mind:

- Pick your time and place (turn off the television).
- Get players in game formation.
- Name the game. State the object in a few simple words.
- Describe the technical details; set the boundaries; demonstrate.
- Give an opportunity for children to ask questions.
- Start the game, modifying where necessary.
- Terminate at the high point—don't play the game too long.
- Retire from leadership. Give the game back to the children.
- Teach another game. Let children return on their own to the ones they enjoy.

Beyond teaching children the favorite games of *your* youth, make physical activity a part of your regular routine. Make it a family affair!

Be active when you take little ones to the park. Push swings and play tag—don't just sit and watch. When appropriate, avoid chauffeuring your children. Encourage them to ride bikes or walk whenever possible. Get them to help with active chores around the house. And go on weekend activity outings when you can—enjoy the outdoors together.

AT SCHOOL

Quality, daily physical education makes perfect sense. Beyond the obvious physical health benefits of regular activity, there are many other reasons why physical education should be a cornerstone of the curriculum in *every* school.

Exercise leads to a state of relaxation, lasting up to two hours, that is accompanied by improved concentration, enhanced creativity and memory, and better task performance and problem solving. In short, physical activity "sets up" students to be ready to learn.

Long-term benefits of physical activity include increased self-confidence and self-image along with decreased anxiety and aggression. In schools with a quality physical education program, these benefits translate into a positive atmosphere and fewer discipline problems.

This improvement in turn leads to enhanced academic performance. A pioneering study done in France in the 1950s demonstrated this. It reduced the time spent on academics and increased that spent on physical education to ensure a quality, daily program. The result? The academic performance, discipline, enthusiasm, fitness, and health of students who participated were superior to those who were not involved. Other studies have shown similar results.

Despite the evidence of its value, quality physical education in the schools is still more a dream than reality. Parents would thus be wise to check on the status at their children's school. Here are some questions to ask:

- Do children get at least 30 minutes of physical education each day?

- Does the program emphasize a fun, social atmosphere and active living rather than just competition and traditional team sports?

- Does your child look forward to participating?

If change is warranted, here are some things you can do:

- *Discuss your concerns.* Meet with the teacher and school administrators. Find out where they stand on the issue. Ask what you can do to help.

- *Get organized.* Develop a parent action group. Generate support. Write the local newspaper.

- *Go to the top if necessary.* Meet with school board officials and politicians responsible for education. Ask for their support *and* action!

ORGANIZED SPORTS AND GAMES

Sports clichés abound in our culture. "Winning isn't everything, it's the only thing" is a well-known call to action. "One hundred and ten percent is not enough" is another good one. Then some sportsmanship-minded idealist came along with "It's not whether you win or lose, it's how you play the game."

What really does matter in sport? Are the values and motives of serious sports played by adults appropriate in sports and games for children and youth?

Research shows that *fun* is a big reason why kids want to participate. The most important factors contributing to the fun of sport are excitement, learning and doing skills, and the opportunity for personal accomplishment.

Next in importance come the social aspects—being on a team, being with friends. Finally, of lesser importance, are winning, getting rewards, and pleasing others. So much for winning being the only thing!

For those who organize sports and games for kids, here are some simple ways to create a friendly, comfortable atmosphere:

- *Focus on skill development.* Improved skills will lead to feelings of satisfaction and accomplishment, which in turn will bring enjoyment and fun.

- *Provide realistic challenges.* Children and youth will learn and grow through a *progressive* series of challenges that are appropriate for their skill level and development. Take things slowly . . . one step at a time.

- *Emphasize personal success.* Playing well, or the feeling that one has played well, is an essential part of the fun of sport. Make a point of complimenting kids both for their effort and for their improvement.

- *Keep winning in perspective.* In the earliest years of organized sport, winning should be a non-issue. (While the kids may try to keep score, the adults don't have to!) As kids get older, being on the winning side should always be less important than simply *striving* to win. By striving to win, kids learn to concentrate, try hard, and be the best they can be!

We must also remember that many children aren't comfortable with competition. It's important to create opportunities for them to enjoy all sorts of activities in a friendly and nonthreatening way.

Regular physical activity and good health habits, planted early, will stand children and youth in good stead as they get older. *All* children deserve a good start. As the booklet *Moving Into the Teens* says, "When it comes to bodies, there's only one per customer."

Sports for Kids

The following comment, by David Gey, first appeared in the December 1976 issue of *The Christian Athlete*. It was wisely reprinted—to make a point—in the book *Joy and Sadness in Children's Sports*. It may be slightly tongue in cheek, but it serves as a strong reminder that organized sports for kids really are for the kids. Whatever role adults play, it should always be encouraging, supportive, and positive.

I believe the youth league idea is a great one with some minor changes: Put an eight-foot board fence around the playing area and only let the kids inside; take away all uniforms and let the kids wear street clothes; let them choose teams by the one po- tato, two potato system; let them play until it gets dark or until the kid with the ball goes home.

SUITING YOURSELF

A big part of active living is doing what's right for you—suiting yourself. Due to personal circumstances, some people may have to be careful about the activities they choose and how they do them. Other people may face limitations that affect their opportunities.

These issues are addressed in the following pages. Common health concerns are considered first, followed by a look at activity and aging, and other challenges. Follow this special advice as needed.

HEALTH CONCERNS

If you have any condition that could be aggravated or complicated by physical activity, take extra caution. If you plan to become *much more* physically active, start by completing the *PAR-Q & YOU* form on page 44. Follow the advice provided there. (A "Yes" response to any PAR-Q question means you are to see your doctor before undertaking any significant increase in activity.)

You might want to discuss with your health care provider any of the following information that is relevant to you. Between the two of you, you can determine the best plan of action. Simply stated: If you have *any* special concerns, then special advice is warranted.

Heart Conditions

Many heart conditions respond positively to regular physical activity. Progressive exercise, in fact, is a central part of rehabilitation programs for many people who have suffered heart attacks. If you have a heart condition, ask your doctor if there are any restrictions or limitations on your being more active. If your doctor *discourages* physical activity, you might want to seek a second opinion.

Bone, Joint, and Muscle Problems

The nature and seriousness of your condition will determine what's suitable for you. If you have arthritis in your knees, for example, swimming or cycling might be a good activity to choose. With your weight supported, these activities are easier on the body. Whatever the concern, perform activities within your limits and listen to the body's pain messages.

Overweight

Those who are excessively overweight (*obese* is the term used in health circles) should take special care in choosing activities, just as those with bone and joint problems must. While the easy rhythm of walking may be just fine, the extra pressure on the joints caused by running could lead to problems. If you're convinced you should be a runner, it might be better to wait until you're a little lighter. (Cycling and swimming are great easy-on-the-joints alternatives.)

Pregnancy

There was a time when women were encouraged to "take it easy" and "keep their feet up" during pregnancy. Attitudes have changed over the years, and regular physical activity during pregnancy is now considered natural and normal. Those who are already active can generally continue with their routines. Others who were inactive before pregnancy may find this an ideal time to start doing a *little bit* more. The key is to participate at a *comfortable* level and take rest breaks regularly. Avoid activities that involve physical contact or danger of falling. Caution is also advised in any situation where the mother's core body temperature can rise (this could happen through strenuous activity or even just sitting in the sun, a sauna, or a hot tub).

AGING ACTIVELY

"How old would you be if you didn't know how old you was?" This question, once posed by the great baseball pitcher Satchel Paige, gets at the heart of how much our *attitude* affects the way we age.

We have tended to accept a gradual physical decline as a natural part of aging. But research now shows that as much as a half of the decline between the ages of 30 and 70 is due not to aging itself but to an inactive way of life.

Regular physical activity keeps bones dense and strong and maintains range of movement in the joints. It also helps maintain balance, coordination, and agility. These all help reduce the risk of falling, a real worry for many older people since falls are a major contributor to reduced mobility and loss of independence.

There are other simple (but important!) benefits. Regular activity helps keep you "regular": It aids digestion and reduces the incidence of constipation. It also provides extra energy and helps you relax and sleep better.

When advising older adults about physical activity, I always remind them that they're not different—just older. That's why I've used this space to highlight some of the benefits of active living (that were extolled at greater length in chapter 1) rather than give detailed specific advice. The many approaches to active living are discussed throughout the book, with special cautions and suggestions noted where appropriate. This information is suitable for everybody, regardless of age.

If you remain active as you get older, you'll have a better chance of living up to the ancient Greek adage that talks of "dying young, at a very old age."

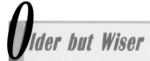
Older but Wiser

For many older people, the obstacles to active living include concerns about physical abilities and the misconception about how much activity is necessary. These needn't be a problem. When it comes to activity and aging:

- Everyone stands to benefit.

- Everyone can do a little more.

- Every little bit helps!

OTHER CHALLENGES

Individuals of *all* ages face special challenges that can affect their opportunities to be active. No matter what the challenge is, rising to meet it will be worth the effort.

Individuals with physical disabilities, for example, stand to benefit from active living in some very special ways:

- Increased strength and flexibility can make daily tasks easier.

- Improved posture helps reduce the aches and pains that can accompany long periods of sitting.

- Better circulation reduces the possibility of blood-pooling and swelling in the legs.

- Maintaining a healthy weight helps those who use wheelchairs (or other mobility aids) to transfer and get around with less effort, making them more mobile.

- Improved stamina and self-confidence can bring greater independence.

In spite of these incentives, many people with disabilities still find it difficult to be active. Obstacles can include lack of information on available programs, inaccessible facilities, transportation problems, and lack of a partner to provide assistance and support. Individuals with physical disabilities aren't the only ones facing these obstacles. Hearing and vision impairments, speaking difficulties, and mental limitations all pose particular demands on those who want to be active.

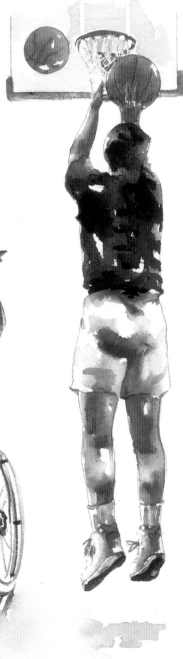

There are things we all can do to help:

- *Individuals with disabilities*. They can focus their attention by evaluating different options and planning ways to overcome *their* obstacles to participation.

- *Leaders*. Those in leadership roles can let individuals make their own decisions about what they can and cannot do. They can also create open and accepting environments and make modifications where appropriate.

- *All of us*. We all can reach out and help others in their efforts to be active. Encouraging and assisting a family member, neighbor, or friend can make the active living experience especially meaningful for both of you.

During his Man-in-Motion tour, Rick Hansen wheeled his chair some 25,000 miles through 34 countries. Along the way, he increased awareness of the barriers that still exist for many who wish to be active, and he encouraged all those he touched to focus on the *abilities* of people with disabilities. It was a gentle reminder that we all have limitations of one sort or another—it's just that some are more visible and severe than others. The important thing is to build on our own abilities and do activities that suit us.

CHAPTER 4

BEYOND THE BASICS

Six Steps to Success

Many modest movers soon find they're interested in a little more. They find they do want to set aside time for an exercise class, regular cycling with friends, or some friendly competition in squash. There are all kinds of activities to discover and enjoy. Each activity—each kind of motion—has its own special rewards. But they are not easily or quickly won. It may take some time (and patience) before you experience the rewards of activity. The Six Steps to Success can help you get there.

STEP #1 laments (and quickly dispenses with) fitness *myth*information.

STEP #2 offers a simple questionnaire to help you decide if you are ready for action.

STEP #3 explains the health components of fitness and how simple it is to improve and maintain them.

STEP #4 provides some tips for starting and persisting.

STEP #5 covers injury prevention and safety.

STEP #6 points you in the right direction if you would like a fitness appraisal or some personal advice.

Use this information as a guide when you explore and experience the activities in chapters 5 and 6 or others of your own choosing.

STEP #1: DISPENSING WITH THE MYTHS

When it comes to quackery, the field of nutrition may lead the way. Unfortunately, the fitness field has its own equivalents of bee pollen and the grapefruit diet. The problem is that as soon as we dispense with one exercise gadget or flaky idea, another one comes along. Let's confront the myths first, then move on to sensible ideas.

DON'T BE DUPED

"Gizmo 812" is my name for the latest item promising miraculous weight loss in no time, a lean, rock-hard body in just days, or great gains in fitness with minimal effort.

Rubber apparel to "sweat off" weight has long been popular with some people. "Jiggly belts" had their day in the sun, too. Toning tables are a more recent addition to the stable of "passive activity" options. Like their predecessors, they have nothing to offer healthy, active adults looking to improve their fitness.

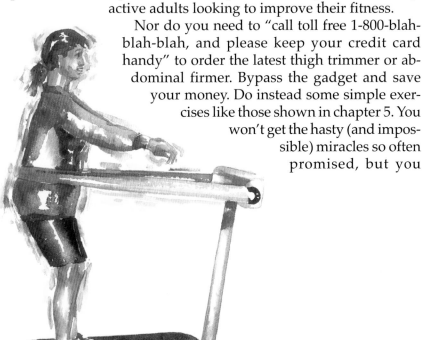

Nor do you need to "call toll free 1-800-blah-blah-blah, and please keep your credit card handy" to order the latest thigh trimmer or abdominal firmer. Bypass the gadget and save your money. Do instead some simple exercises like those shown in chapter 5. You won't get the hasty (and impossible) miracles so often promised, but you will see change and improvement you can realistically expect for your effort.

In commenting on the never-ending stream of exercise gimmicks, gadgets, and gizmos, *Consumer Reports* said, quite simply, "If something sounds too good to be true, it probably is."

When it comes to fitness, you can't get something for nothing. And you don't always get what you pay for.

FORGET THE FOLKLORE

Along with the gadgets, all sorts of strange notions have worked their way into our fitness consciousness. "No pain, no gain" is a long-standing pest. (It ranks right up there with "110% is not enough.") The only response to this maxim is "no way"—*easy does it!*

Special potions to rid the body of "cellulite" (a nonsense name for fat), the idea that muscle turns to fat if you stop strength training, and the ever-popular concept of spot reduction (doing exercises to lose weight and fat in certain places) are *not* supported by scientific research. Forget about them. If you're eating properly, you don't need protein or other food supplements when you're exercising vigorously. Also, there is no perfect activity. Nor is there a perfect time of day to exercise. There are lots of other claims about exercise and fitness that we don't need and aren't true.

What *is* needed is some straightforward information and advice. So, on to Step #2.

STEP #2: ASSESSING YOUR READINESS

Some people starting a vigorous activity program jump right in. Others feel that they should have some sort of test or see their doctor first.

Fortunately, there is another choice: *PAR-Q & You*—the *Physical Activity Readiness Questionnaire*—will help you decide if you are ready to go. Here's how to proceed:

- Read it carefully.
- Answer the questions.
- Follow the "yes" or "no" advice, whichever applies to you.

PAR-Q & YOU
(A Questionnaire for People Aged 15 to 69)

Regular physical activity is fun and healthy, and increasingly more people are starting to become more active every day. Being more active is very safe for most people. However, some people should check with their doctors before they start becoming much more physically active.

If you are planning to become much more physically active than you are now, start by answering the seven questions below. If you are between the ages of 15 and 69, the PAR-Q will tell you if you should check with your doctor before you start. If you are over 69 years of age, and you are not used to being very active, check with your doctor.

Common sense is your best guide when you answer these questions. Please read the questions carefully and answer each one honestly: Check YES or NO.

YES NO

❑ ❑ 1. Has your doctor ever said that you have a heart condition *and* that you should only do physical activity recommended by a doctor?

❑ ❑ 2. Do you feel pain in your chest when you do physical activity?

❑ ❑ 3. In the past month, have you had chest pain when you were not doing physical activity?

❑ ❑ 4. Do you lose your balance because of dizziness or do you ever lose consciousness?

❑ ❑ 5. Do you have a bone or joint problem that could be made worse by a change in your physical activity?

❑ ❑ 6. Is your doctor currently prescribing drugs (for example, water pills) for your blood pressure or heart condition?

❑ ❑ 7. Do you know of <u>any other reason</u> why you should not do physical activity?

If you answered YES to one or more questions

Talk with your doctor by phone or in person BEFORE you start becoming much more physically active or BEFORE you have a fitness appraisal. Tell your doctor about the PAR-Q and which questions you answered YES.

- You may be able to do any activity you want—as long as you start slowly and build up gradually. Or, you may need to restrict your activities to those that are safe for you. Talk with your doctor about the kinds of activities you wish to participate in and follow his/her advice.
- Find out which community programs are safe and helpful for you.

If you answered NO to all questions

If you answered NO honestly to all PAR-Q questions, you can be reasonably sure that you can

- start becoming much more physically active—begin slowly and build up gradually. This is the safest and easiest way to go.
- take part in a fitness appraisal—this is an excellent way to determine your basic fitness so that you can plan the best way for you to live actively. (For more on this see pp. 57-62.)

DELAY BECOMING MUCH MORE ACTIVE:

- if you are not feeling well because of a temporary illness such as a cold or a fever—wait until you feel better; or
- if you are or may be pregnant—talk to your doctor before you start becoming more active.

Please note: If your health changes so that you then answer YES to any of the above questions, tell your fitness or health professional. Ask whether you should change your physical activity plan.

STEP #3: STRIVING FOR TOTAL FITNESS

Fitness has three important components: *stamina, suppleness,* and *strength.* Call them the 3 Ss if you like. Any exercise program worth the time and effort should address all three.

Body composition is a fourth component. You can possess great stamina, suppleness, and strength, but you're not *totally* healthy and fit if you're overweight. Excessive weight increases the risk of a number of conditions, including heart disease, high blood pressure, and diabetes. Weight loss is a consuming passion for many people, but it needn't be. Follow the tips for healthy eating (in chapter 7) and active living (throughout the book) and you can achieve *and* maintain a *healthy* body weight.

STAMINA

Stamina is your distance from fatigue. It's a simple word meaning the same as cardiovascular endurance. It has to do with how easily your lungs take in oxygen and how efficiently your heart pumps the oxygen-rich blood to your various body parts and internal organs. Having sufficient stamina means tiring less quickly in anything you do, and it offers other important benefits.

Activities performed at a moderate-intensity level help to develop stamina. Indoors this could mean participating along with your favorite television exercise show or video, jumping rope, or using exercise equipment. Outdoors you can turn to walking, running, cycling, or a host of other enjoyable activities. For any aerobic/endurance activity, you can't go wrong if you follow the FITT formula.

The *intensity* part of the FITT formula suffers by far the most from abuse. The inaccurate "no pain, no gain" philosophy has led many to think that if you don't finish your session huffing, puffing, red in the face, and looking for the nearest couch, then you didn't go hard enough.

"Easy does it" *is* the way to go, especially if you're just getting into a vigorous activity program. There are three simple *pacing techniques* to help you make sure you don't overdo.

- *The Talk Test.* This method, popularized years ago by Bill Bowerman when he was the University of Oregon track coach, encourages you to move along at a conversation pace. If you

The FITT* Formula

- *F* is for *frequency*. Start with three days a week (or every other day). Add more days later if you wish and when you're ready for them.

- *I* is for **intensity**. Go at a *pace* that's just right for *you*: not too fast, not too slow. Check the pacing techniques in this chapter, and try one as a guide.

- *T* is for **time**. Start with fifteen to twenty minutes of *moving*. Depending on your activity, you can "work" and "rest" (go faster, then slower). Build up to fifteen minutes of *continuous* activity, then gradually extend the length of your sessions. These longer bouts of activity improve cardiovascular endurance.

- *T* is for **type**. Activity choices are almost endless. Some are described in chapters 5 and 6; others appear on the active living list in chapter 2. You can add to these. Whatever you choose, do activities you enjoy and that bring you some satisfaction.

*FITT acronym courtesy of David M. Chisholm, MD.

can't talk when you're exercising, you're going too fast. (*Not* recommended when swimming!)

- *The Feel Test.* This method suggests going by how you feel. It's based on the Ratings of Perceived Exertion scale developed by Swedish physiologist G.A. Borg. The scale has intensity ratings from very, very light to very, very hard. Borg recommends you exercise at a comfortable level, somewhere between fairly light and somewhat hard.

- *The Pulse Test*. This method involves counting your pulse (also known as heart-rate monitoring). You can use the *Heart Rate Target Zone* chart as a guide; it shows age along the bottom and pulse rate (in beats per 10 seconds) along the side.

The target zone is determined first by establishing the *predicted maximum* heart rate for each age. (The number that is commonly used is 220 minus the age in years.) The bottom of the green zone in the chart is then set at 55% of the age-predicted maximum heart rate. Any activity that raises your pulse to this level or higher is considered *moderate intensity*. Activities that get the pulse into the green zone bring with them significant health benefits, primarily in the form of reduced risk of coronary heart disease.

If you want to improve your cardiovascular fitness, strive to work at a level that gets your pulse into the yellow zone, raising it to at least 70% of your age-predicted maximum. If you're just beginning, aim to be at or near the lower end of this zone.

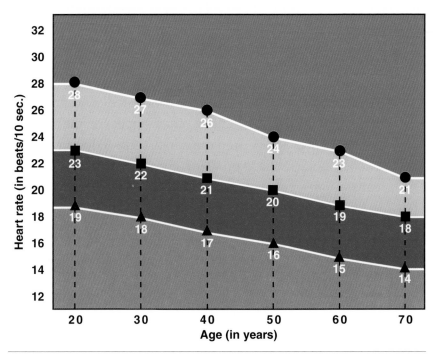

The Canadian Society for Exercise Physiology uses 55% of the age-predicted maximum heart rate as the lower limit for moderate-intensity activity. The American College of Sports Medicine uses 60%. For practical purposes, this difference is insignificant.

Use the pulse rates shown in the chart as a *guide,* not as firm numbers cast in stone. For example, the chart may be inappropriate for cardiac patients and individuals on certain heart medications. Depending on your genetic inheritance, your own maximum heart rate could be as much as 10% above or below the predicted maximum (which is really just an average). So if you find your heart rate is near the lower end of the yellow zone when you're active but it still feels too demanding, slow down to a more comfortable pace. You'll still be in the green zone and reaping important health benefits. You can up the tempo gradually as you progress with your program.

Pulse Counting

To count your pulse accurately:

- Use the index and middle fingers. Place them gently on the inside of the wrist just below the thumb or on the side of the neck just behind the Adam's apple.

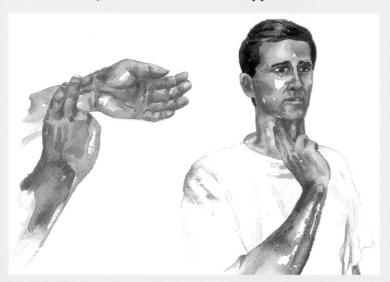

- Count for ten seconds, starting five seconds after you stop exercising. Count the first pulse as "0" (that is, count 0, 1, 2, 3 . . .).

The talk test, the feel test, and the pulse test are great in the *early* stages of a program. After a while you'll have a natural feel for how fast you want to go and you won't need to use them anymore.

SUPPLENESS

Suppleness (or flexibility) allows you to bend, turn, and reach with ease and comfort. It plays a part in maintaining proper posture, reduces stiffness and soreness from unaccustomed activity, and helps minimize the risk of back injury.

Regular bending and stretching movements that take the muscles and joints through their full range can improve (and then maintain) flexibility. Indoors, a simple stretching routine will accomplish this. (*Stretch It* on pp. 65-70 is a good starter program. Be sure to follow the *Principles for Stretching* given here when you do it or any similar routine.) Yoga and Tai Chi offer similar benefits and other rewards as well. Outdoor activities like gardening and yard work can help you stay flexible, too.

*P**rinciples for Stretching*

To experience the benefits of a stretching routine:

- Stretch slowly and smoothly without bouncing or jerking.

- Use gentle, continuous movement or stretch-and-hold, whichever is right for the exercise.

- Strive for a stretched, relaxed feeling. Avoid pain—it means you're stretching too far.

- Don't hold your breath. Breathe in a natural rhythm.

- Start with several repetitions of each exercise.

- For stretch-and-hold exercises, start by holding each repetition for a minimum of 10 seconds. Later, do fewer repetitions, but hold each one longer (15 or 20 seconds, for example).

- Avoid exercises that hurt or feel uncomfortable.

STRENGTH

The strength you need isn't the "you too can get big biceps and kick sand in somebody's face" variety. It's merely sufficient strength to contribute to proper posture and to let you accomplish daily tasks without difficulty.

Exercises and activities that tax the muscles a little beyond their normal capacity help to improve strength and muscular endurance. Indoors this can come from a simple calisthenics routine (like *Strength Fit* on pp. 70-74) on through to strength training programs using special equipment. Outdoors, all sorts of activities will do it. Heavy yard work, chores around the house, raking and carrying leaves, and shoveling snow are everyday activities that can do their part to develop and maintain your strength.

Strength training with weights—once the domain of weightlifters, bodybuilders, and serious athletes—is now a popular fitness activity. With this popularity has come a profusion of programs, many of them much more complicated than they need to be. (Physical educator Arthur Steinhaus had a great answer for those who were bent on making a program overly sophisticated. "If you want to get strong," he'd say, "play tiddlywinks. But use manhole covers.")

Strength training with equipment *can* be simple. Use a good (simple!) book or booklet as your guide, or get some instruction from a fitness specialist at a nearby facility. And follow these *Steps to Strength* as you pursue your program:

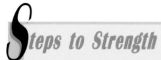

teps to Strength

For strength training with weights:

- Warm up well at the beginning of each session.

- Learn proper technique. Protect your back and joints from undue stress.

- Build muscular endurance. Use light weights and high repetitions (two to four sets of ten to fifteen or more repetitions of each exercise).

(continued)

- Inhale and exhale on each repetition, exhaling on effort.

- Take a brief rest between sets—a minute or so, just enough time to catch your breath.

- Avoid exercises that hurt or feel uncomfortable.

- Keep a training record. It can be very motivating, and it promotes progress.

- Vary your routine to keep things interesting.

STEP #4: STICKING WITH YOUR PROGRAM

The road to a more active lifestyle is paved with good intentions and littered with dropouts. Most people *want* to be more active. And lots of individuals do find ways to include physical activity during their leisure time. But far too many don't stick with their plans.

There are some things you can do to increase the odds in your favor. Start by reviewing the list of "obstacles" in *Overcoming Inactivity*. Check (✓) the ones that apply to you. Keep these in mind as you consider the starting and persisting tips in this section as well as the suggestions in steps #5 and #6. All this advice is to help you get through the period when you may be active because you feel you *should* be—and on to the time when you are because you *want* to be.

OVERCOMING INACTIVITY—THE TEN LACKS

Research has identified a number of obstacles, real or perceived, to starting *or* staying with a leisure-time physical activity program. The important ones—the "Ten Lacks"—appear here.

Lack of . . .

- [ ] ability
- [ ] energy
- [ ] facilities
- [ ] family support
- [ ] interest

- [ ] money
- [ ] motivation
- [ ] partners
- [ ] self-discipline
- [ ] time

If some of these obstacles are *your* obstacles, use the suggestions throughout the rest of this chapter to help you overcome them. If (when!) you succeed, you may find yourself saying, "Those weren't obstacles at all, I was just making excuses!"

STARTING

Consider these suggestions *before* you go to your first class, swim your first lap, or play your first game. They'll help get you off to a good start.

- *Set some goals.* Your goals should be relevant and realistic for you. If you like short-term goals (weekly, for example), they should focus on such things as the number of activity sessions you complete. Longer term goals (six weeks or more) could involve fitness improvement, weight lost, number of repetitions, and the like. Write your goals down, and refer to them regularly to see how you're doing.

- *Keep records.* Use a little book or a calendar to keep track of what you do. (This is a perfect place to list your goals, too.) Recording your activity sessions can remind you of days missed, and it offers tangible evidence of progress.

- *Establish a routine.* Pick a time of day that suits your schedule. Morning, afternoon, or evening, it really doesn't matter. The best time of day is the one that's right for you. Experiment and find a comfortable routine.

- *Avoid hassles.* Some activities are more accessible than others. You can walk, run, or cycle right from your front door. Swimming or an activity class may not be so convenient. Make sure your activity interests you enough that you will accept the travel time or any inconveniences that may occur.

- *Participate with friends.* Physical activity can provide opportunities to enjoy the company of others. If you like this social side, you could join a club, take a class, or get involved in other group activities. If you like a less structured approach, you can participate with your family, neighbors, or friends.

- *Don't rush.* Set aside enough time for your activity. Appointments or other commitments pressing your session can make you a clock watcher and spoil much of what physical activity has to offer. Remember, your activity is supposed to be your *re-creation.* Finish relaxed and refreshed.

PERSISTING

Once you've launched into a program, the challenge is to stay with it. Here are some tips to help.

- *Don't get down.* It's natural to miss sessions from time to time. Work or family responsibilities sometimes get in the way. And if you're tired, it's sometimes better to take a day off. When you do miss a session, just start planning for your next outing—don't feel as though you have failed this time.

- *Make activity a family affair.* The encouragement and support of your family is particularly important. Their acceptance of your desire for more physical activity is important, so it helps if you can be active together. Then you can pull each other along on days you don't feel quite up to it.

- *Avoid boredom.* Routines are good, but when you get into a rut it's time for a change. Boredom is self-inflicted. Don't be a slave to any program. Make some changes when necessary and your activity will be fun again.

- *Use rewards.* Rewards help some people persist, so use them if they work for you. Remember how much fun it was as a kid to save up for something special, then finally go out and get it? You can follow the same idea here. When you achieve goals you have set, treat yourself to something you wouldn't normally do or buy.

- *Lose weight, not heart.* If you're trying to lose some weight, don't despair, and don't feel you need to be *solely* concerned with weight loss. Remember that activity increases muscle tone, so you may be gaining muscle while losing fat and inches. Your *weight* may not decrease significantly, but your body *shape* may improve. Consult your mirror and check the fit of your clothes, while monitoring the scale for signs of positive change.

- *Be patient.* Don't rush or force things. Look for improvement over the long term, not overnight.

One final bit of advice—*have fun!* An activity that is sheer boredom and punishment for one individual may be pure delight to another. If you are utterly convinced you're not a runner, for example, then don't run to get fit. Choose activities that you are comfortable with and that suit your disposition—ones that you feel will bring you some enjoyment and satisfaction.

Keep in mind, too, that your interests may change over time. I remember a former military type who at first reveled in the hard calisthenics issued by his fitness instructor. But later he came to enjoy slow runs and yoga. So as *you* enjoy your activities, be open to experimenting and to trying new things.

STEP #5: PLAYING IT SAFE

The best advice I can give about injuries is this: *Don't get them!* Chapters 5 and 6 discuss injury prevention and safety relative to the activities covered there. Each activity has its own particular demands that require special attention. Heed the advice provided, and you're well on your way to enjoyable, injury-free activity. This step offers more general advice on injury prevention and for dealing with injuries when they do occur.

INJURY PREVENTION

A relaxed attitude and realistic approach to physical activity can go a long way toward preventing injuries. Here are a few suggestions:

- *Exercise regularly.* Your activity should be regular and moderate, not sporadic and intense. For most of the activities in chapters 5 and 6, a routine of three times a week or every other day (as suggested earlier in the FITT formula) is the best way to start.

- *Take it easy.* Endurance activities—indoor cycling, swimming, running, and the like—should be vigorous, but not *too* demanding. The pacing techniques on pages 46-50 can help you make sure you're not going at it too hard.

- *Be your own boss.* Some programs (like TV exercise shows or videotapes) will encourage you to go at a certain rate. If it's too fast, slow down. If any exercises or activities are uncomfortable, stop doing them. (You'd then be wise to find a fitness specialist who can check your technique to see if this is the problem.) The point here is that activity is an *individual* thing. Do what's *best* for you.

- *Don't overdo it.* Your activity should increase your energy level, not reduce it; it ought to make you feel better, not worse. If you have a feeling of tiredness that lingers after your session, difficulty sleeping, or a buildup of fatigue, you're doing too much. Other signs of overdoing it include an increase of five to ten beats in your normal resting heart rate, unexplained weight loss, and an increased frequency of sore throats and colds. Experiment and find the amount of activity that's just right for you.

INJURY CARE AND TREATMENT

If in spite of all precautions you sustain an injury, this is what you should do:

- *Act fast.* Responding immediately—whether it's to a muscle strain, a joint injury, or a blow from a racquet or ball—can help minimize damage and speed recovery. See *RICE It* for the steps to take.

- *Seek medical advice when necessary.* Minor injuries may respond to self-treatment. More serious or persistent problems will require medical attention. When you do get medical advice, follow it. Don't let things get worse through lack of proper care.

- *Take corrective action.* Injury can result from inadequate footwear or improper equipment. It can also be caused by biomechanical abnormalities, such as high arches or flat feet. And it can result from strength or flexibility imbalances. If any of these causes is identified, corrective action can be taken. (A sports medicine specialist could be a big help here.)

For injury prevention *and* proper recovery after injury, *be sensible!* One physician quoted in a *Time* article on sports injuries said that too many of those who get injured suffer from what he calls "an acute case of simplemindedness." They try for too much, too soon. And they don't listen to their bodies.

It's good to be enthusiastic and enjoy your activity. But it's important to balance your enthusiasm with good sense.

R ICE It

For immediate treatment of joint and muscle injuries:

*R*est the injured body part.

*I*ce the injured body part (for 10-20 minutes every few hours).

*C*ompress the injured area with an elastic bandage or towel if swelling occurs.

*E*levate the injured area above heart level.

STEP #6: TESTING YOUR FITNESS, GETTING ADVICE

Curious about your current level of fitness? If so, you might want to have a formal fitness appraisal done or try the do-it-yourself one provided here. I say "might want to" because, while an appraisal can be helpful, it shouldn't be considered mandatory for starting a formal activity program.

An initial fitness appraisal followed by another one some weeks into the program can be very motivating for some people but do little to inspire others. If you feel this will help you stick with *your* routine, consider it part of your motivational repertoire, along with the starting and persisting tips in Step #4.

If you want specific advice to help you develop a program or if you have other questions or concerns, a qualified fitness specialist can be a big help. Professionals at recreation centers, YMCAs and YWCAs, clubs, universities and colleges, and other facilities can administer your fitness appraisal (if you want one) *and* provide informal advice.

APPRAISAL AND ADVICE

Fitness appraisals can range from simple and inexpensive to complex and costly. Most appraisals assess your cardiovascular endurance (stamina), strength and muscular endurance, flexibility, and body composition. Some appraisals consider additional health habits, as discussed in chapter 7.

This information (showing areas that may deserve particular attention) is used along with your activity interests, current activity pattern, and hopes for change to develop a realistic and meaningful plan of action. This initial appraisal also provides a benchmark to help chart your progress. A *less formal approach* may not include a professionally administered appraisal but can be helpful nonetheless. Your fitness specialist can answer pressing questions and offer simple tips and advice to spur you on and help keep you on track. Whichever approach you prefer, it's important to consult someone with the training, skills, and experience to guide you properly. See pages 123-124 for further details.

DO-IT-YOURSELF APPRAISAL

If you're so inclined, there are some simple ways to check your progress.

For *stamina*, think about the activities you're doing. If after a while you're swimming farther without having to stop for a rest, your cardiovascular fitness is improving. The same goes if you are coming on strong at the end of your game of racquetball or tennis when your opponent is starting to fade. Comparable changes in other activities demonstrate similar improvement.

For *suppleness*, you can use the exercises in the *Stretch It* routine (see pp. 65-70) as a guide. As time goes on, if you are stretching farther comfortably you're improving.

DO-IT-YOURSELF FITNESS APPRAISAL

In this appraisal you're not measuring yourself against some predetermined standard. Personal improvement is what you are after! Compare your results from one appraisal to the next to see how you're doing.

	Appraisal #1	Appraisal #2	Appraisal #3
	Date:_____	Date:_____	Date:_____
Fitness component			
Stamina			
Endurance activity:			
_____	_____	_____	_____
Suppleness			
Forward stretch	_____	_____	_____
Strength and muscular endurance			
Push-up	_____	_____	_____
	(max 30)	(max 30)	(max 30)
Curl-up	_____	_____	_____
	(max 30)	(max 30)	(max 30)

For *strength and muscular endurance,* use the exercises in the *Strength Fit* routine (see pp. 70-74) as a measure. Over time, if you're naturally doing more repetitions, you're getting stronger.

For *body composition,* use the full-length-mirror test or the fit-of-your-clothes test as mentioned on page 55. For more detailed techniques of assessing body composition, see a fitness specialist.

If you want to be a little more precise, try the *Do-It-Yourself Fitness Appraisal.* You can use the form provided here to record your results, or reproduce it in your activity journal if you are keeping one.

Here are some tips to help you with your appraisal:

First Appraisal

In the column for Appraisal #1, write down the date you're doing it, then enter your results as you complete each item. When you've done this appraisal, you will have your benchmark. When you do Appraisal #2, you can compare your results and check for improvement.

Stamina

Pick your favorite endurance activity—walking, cycling, swimming, in-line skating, you name it. Find a measured course (running track, swimming pool, etc.) or measure one yourself using a car odometer. Then get moving, and go as far as you can in fifteen minutes. Record your result.

Be careful not to overdo. If you haven't done this sort of activity before, your tendency may be to start out too quickly. Go at a steady, comfortable pace. You can always increase the tempo if you're feeling really strong near the end.

When you do your follow-up appraisal, try for a greater distance in fifteen minutes, or try to go the distance you achieved in the first appraisal in less time. Record your result and compare—farther or faster and you're getting better!

Suppleness

As a warm-up, do four stretches (two with each leg) as shown in Exercise 4 on page 67. Hold each stretch for ten to fifteen seconds. For the appraisal, do the stretch as shown below. Do it twice—using a yardstick or tape measure to record how far you can reach—and write down your best result. (Remember to use a *gentle* stretch-and-hold approach—don't bounce!)

FORWARD STRETCH

This stretch gives a good indication of the suppleness in your lower back and the upper-back part of your legs (the hamstring muscles).

Sit with both legs straight in front, feet slightly apart, and resting against a small bench (turned on its side) or a board. Place the yard-stick or tape measure across the board with the 25-centimeter (or 10-inch) mark even with the feet. With fingers outstretched, reach as far along the stick or tape as you can. Hold, then measure. Don't let the knees bend as you stretch.

Strength and Muscular Endurance

For the two strength items of the appraisal, do as many repetitions of each one as you *comfortably* can—that is, without straining or hold-ing your breath—up to a maximum of thirty. (Even if you can do more, thirty repetitions will demonstrate adequate levels of strength in these muscle groups.) Take five or six minutes of rest between the two tests. Record the number of repetitions you do for each one.

PUSH-UP
This tests the strength and muscular endurance in your shoulders, arms, and chest.

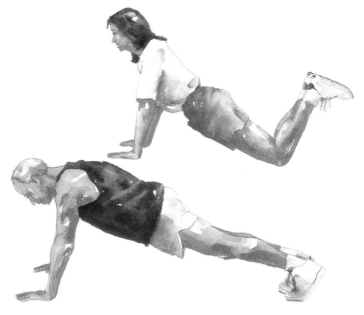

See Exercise 1 in the *Strength Fit* routine on page 71 for the proper technique and procedure.

PARTIAL CURL-UP

This tests the strength and muscular endurance in your abdominal (stomach) muscles.

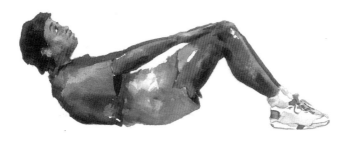

See Exercise 2 in the *Strength Fit* routine on page 71 for the proper technique and procedure. Use the hand / arm position shown in the illustration, sliding your hands up your thighs as far as your knees before returning to the starting position.

Follow-Up Appraisals

Wait at least six or eight weeks before you do Appraisal #2 (ten or twelve weeks would be even better). Allow the same length of time between Appraisals #2 and #3 if you want to assess yourself again. Enter the date of each appraisal and your results in the appropriate column. Compare the results to your previous appraisal.

It's great to see improvement in a fitness appraisal, but what's really important is the *carry-over effect*. Does improvement in your fitness affect your daily routine? Are your normal tasks accomplished with greater ease and comfort? Do you have more energy? Are you less tired at the end of the day?

I still remember a conversation I had many years ago with a participant in a program I was managing. He observed that he always used to stop and rest at the top of a long set of stairs between his garage and house. After a couple of months of regular cycling, he said, "On Saturday, I climbed the stairs with my two-year-old daughter in one arm, a bag of potatoes in the other. I got into the house before it dawned on me I had climbed the stairs and wasn't the least bit out of breath." Active living rewards you in these small, but meaningful, ways.

CHAPTER
5

INDOORS
Exercise, Fun, & Games

This chapter covers what you need to know to get started in a variety of indoor activities. It includes three sections:

- *EXERCISING AT HOME* is the first choice of many. It's comfortable and convenient, and the conditions are ideal (no rain, snow, or darkness to contend with). You'll find a forty-minute starter program along with stretching and strengthening exercises designed for building fitness in your family room. The tips and advice on exercise equipment and resources will help you devise a program that's right for you.

- *CHOOSING A CLASS OR FACILITY* can be challenging. The suggestions provided can help you assess your choices with proper care and attention.

- *PLAYING COURT SPORTS OR TEAM GAMES* is for those who like action and competition. The guidelines for injury prevention and safety will help keep you playing.

EXERCISING AT HOME

Home exercise programs should work on stamina, suppleness, and strength—the 3 Ss of fitness described in chapter 4. If you choose a TV exercise show or video—and it's a *good* one—it will offer a *complete* routine.

If you're devising your own program, you'll have to ensure this completeness yourself. Choose and use exercise equipment wisely, and follow a logical plan. (Why not try the Forty-Minute Starter Program?) Here are a few more suggestions:

- Pick a time of day that suits your schedule, then stick to it.
- Ease into your program. Don't look for quick results.
- Exercise with a friend or neighbor if it will help you stay with it.
- Change your routine from time to time for variety and interest.

Home Exercise: Forty-Minute Starter Program

A good program includes *five* elements:

Warm-up: Two to three minutes. *Easy* endurance activity—walking around (don't worry, no one's watching), stationary cycling, rowing. You decide!

Suppleness: Ten minutes of the *Stretch It* routine (pp. 65-70) or something similar.

Stamina: Fifteen minutes "moving" using the equipment and activity or activities of your choice. Review the FITT formula (p. 47) if you need to.

Strength: Eight to ten minutes of the *Strength Fit* routine (pp. 70-74) or equivalent. You can shorten this segment by eliminating exercises for muscles that are strengthened during the Stamina portion (for example, the Single-Leg Squat can go if you cycled).

Cool-down: Two to three minutes of easy stretching. Do exercises that stretch out the muscles most used during the Stamina part of your session.

*E*xercise Care and Caution

Go gently when you're doing suppleness and strength exercises. Avoid movements that feel uncomfortable or hurt. (Have an exercise specialist check to see if your technique might be the problem.) If you are under the care of a health professional for any muscular or joint problem, do only those exercises and movements you have been instructed to perform.

*S*TRETCH IT

Follow the *Principles for Stretching* (p. 50) when doing this routine.

- Exercise 1 is gentle continuous movement; all the others are stretch-and-hold.

- The descriptions tell you the proper movement. Make sure you repeat the movement on both sides of the body to ensure a balanced routine.

- If you're pressed for time and anxious to get at your game or go for a run, do at least the *Fast Five:* 4, 7, 8, 9, and 10.

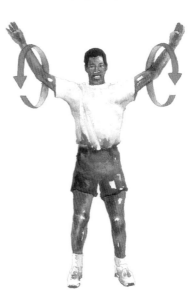

1. ARM CIRCLES
Do full, slow sweeping circles
with both arms—
circle forward, then backward

2. SIDE STRETCH
Reach one arm overhead
and the other down the
side of the leg.

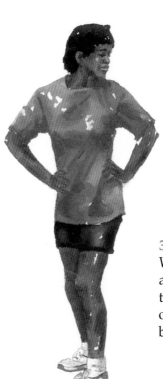

3. TRUNK TWIST
With knees slightly bent
and hands on hips,
trunk twist slowly in
one direction, looking
behind and exhaling.

4. SIT-REACH

With one leg straight and the other bent with the sole of the foot near knee of straight leg, reach out along the straight leg.

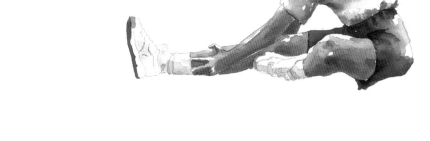

5. PELVIC TILT

Lying on your back, with knees bent and feet flat on the floor, tighten abdominals and buttocks, and press your lower back firmly against the floor.

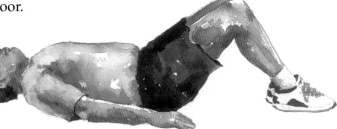

6. SIDE-TO-SIDE
Sit with your legs in front, knees bent and feet flat on the floor. Roll your legs to one side toward the floor, looking over the other shoulder.

7. LOW BACK STRETCH FAST 5
Lying on your back, grasp your hands behind one knee and bring it toward your chest.

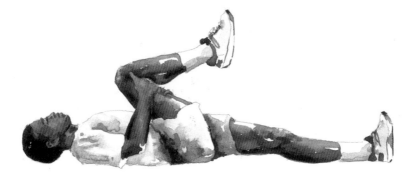

8. SPLIT STRETCH

Stand with legs a little more than shoulder-width apart, feet pointing straight ahead. Shift your weight to the side over one leg, with the other leg kept straight and both feet flat on floor.

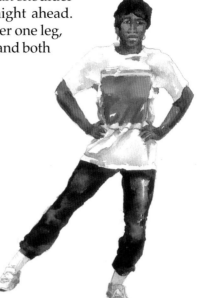

9. THIGH STRETCH

While standing, bend one knee, grasp your ankle, and pull your foot gently toward your buttocks. Keep the supporting leg slightly bent and your back flat. Use a chair for support if you need to.

10. CALF STRETCH

FAST 5

Standing with one foot a little in front of the other
and feet pointing straight ahead, bend both knees (squatting) to
stretch the muscle in the lower part of the rear leg. Repeat with legs
farther apart and back
leg straight to stretch
the calf muscle.

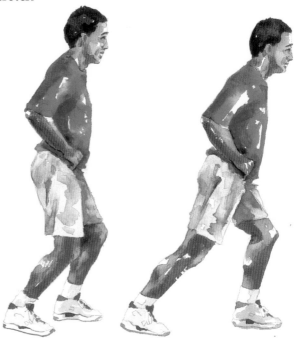

STRENGTH FIT

Review the *Steps to Strength* on pages 51-52 for some safety tips.

- Start with one set of ten repetitions of each exercise. Do this for a few sessions to ease into your routine and learn proper technique. After this, gradually increase your repetitions and sets.

- Once you're doing two or more sets, you can do the routine faster if you do it as a "circuit." That is, do the first set of Exercise 1, the first set of Exercise 2, and so on through to Exercise 6. Then circle back to 1 and go through the sequence again.

- For exercises that work on one side (or leg) at a time, be sure to do the same number of repetitions on each side to ensure a balanced routine.

1. PUSH-UP

Lying on your front, position your hands at shoulder level with palms flat on the floor slightly more than shoulder-width apart. Use either the knees or the feet for a pivot point (whichever is right for you now—using the feet requires more strength). Then, keeping your body in line (don't sag!), straighten your arms to push the body up, then lower it again until you're almost touching the floor.

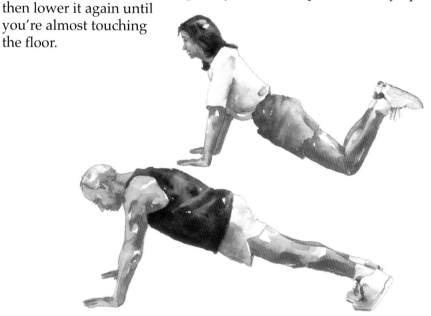

2. PARTIAL CURL-UP

Lie on your back, with knees bent (to about 90°) and feet flat on the floor. Do a "pelvic tilt," pressing your lower back to the floor, then slowly curl forward, lifting your shoulder blades and upper back off the floor. Hold this "up position" for a couple of seconds, then slowly curl back down. Look toward the ceiling (not at your knees) throughout so you don't bend your neck too far forward. Make the curl-up increasingly difficult by progressing through the four arm positions listed. Use whichever method is right for you now, then move on in the progression when you're ready:

- With arms straight, slide hands along the floor.
- With arms straight, slide hands up the thighs as far as the knees.
- Cross arms on the chest.
- Bend arms and hold hands against the ears.

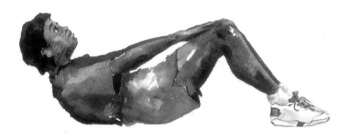

Avoid anchoring your feet down (this reduces the demands on your abdominal muscles), and *avoid* doing curl-ups with your legs straight (this puts undue stress on your lower back).

3. SIDE LEG RAISE
Lying on one side with your head resting on your forearm, raise the top leg slowly, keeping the knee slightly bent and toes pointing toward the floor. Then return to the starting position.

4. ARM CURL

Stand with your knees slightly bent and your back straight. Arms hang down, palms facing forward and the sides of the hands against the thighs. Bend your elbows, curling the arms until the hands reach the shoulders. Then return to the starting position. Hold food cans or other light weights in your hands later to make it more difficult if you like.

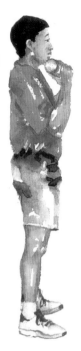

5. SINGLE-LEG SQUAT

Stand with one leg straight and the other bent, the foot held up off the floor and behind. Squat, bending the knee slightly. Use a chair for balance if you need to.

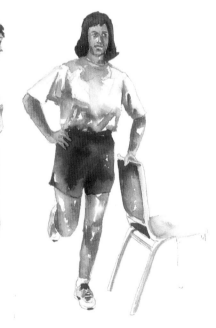

6. CALF RAISE

Stand with feet shoulder-width apart. Raise up on the toes, bending your knees slightly, then lower your heels to the floor again. As you progress, you may want to do the exercise without touching the heels to the floor between repetitions.

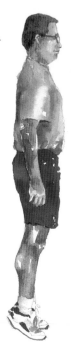

TV EXERCISE SHOWS AND VIDEOTAPES

Exercise shows and videos vary tremendously in style, content, and quality. Some offer a parade of female "models." Others focus so much on abdominal exercises, "toning," and "firming" that you'd think they were training videos for *Hard Bodies III*.

But there are sensible, well-rounded programs and videos, too. To find a good one, follow these guidelines:

- Get advice from a local fitness specialist. Ask someone you respect who is sensitive to your needs.
- Check the qualifications of the instructors. They should be certified by a recognized fitness organization.
- Look for programs that include safe and conservative exercises and encourage you to go at a reasonable pace.
- Try to find resources that educate along with the exercise.
- Borrow or rent videos to try them before you buy them.

*F*amous Fitness

It seems like every second media star has a fitness video (or an audiotape in the early years)—at one time, even Miss Piggy was into it! (Her program promised "no getting out of breath, no messing up your clothes, and no smart-de-pants lectures on 'bad foods.' ") Hers was a spoof, of course, but others are supposed to be serious. If *you're* serious, go beyond the personality and look at the qualifications of the instructor.

EXERCISE EQUIPMENT

We go through all sorts of fads and fashions in our exercise programs and equipment. Though it seems as if stationary bicycles have always been with us, new items join an ever-more-crowded field. Certain pieces of equipment long used in particular sports are "discovered" by the fitness movement and, through it, gain popularity and broader use. Elastic tubing from swimming, the medicine ball from track and field, the slide board from speed skating, and, of course, the rowing ergometer from rowing are just a few examples.

Equipment varies in cost, type, and complexity. Some items are free—you can improvise with food cans and telephone books as light weights for developing strength and muscular endurance. Elastic bands and tubing are inexpensive yet also effective for strengthening via stretch-resistance exercises. Big-ticket items could cost as much as a nice vacation. Some equipment (like a jump rope) is small and portable; other equipment (like a home gym) can fill the corner of a room. Some items develop stamina; others emphasize strength. Many provide a nice combination of the two.

Price is important when you're purchasing, but more important is that the equipment you buy meet your *needs.* If you lean toward higher quality equipment, you will get value for your money. It will be durable and serve you well. Quality equipment will also command a higher resale price if you want to change activities later.

The *problem* for some people with buying exercise equipment is that boredom sets in. What starts as a nice routine soon becomes a rut. But this needn't be the case if equipment is chosen wisely and used well. For help with this, check *Exercise Equipment Options* for the range of possibilities, then heed the advice on choosing it and using it.

Exercise Equipment Options

Major Equipment	Minor Equipment
Cross-country ski machines	Elastic bands and tubing
Exercise bicycles	Food cans and telephone books
Free weights (barbells and dumbbells)	Hand and wrist weights
Home gyms (for strength training)	Jump ropes
Rowing machines	Light dumbbell sets
Stairclimbers	Slide boards
Treadmills	Steps
	Weight belts and bands.

Choosing It

Here are some tips for choosing the "right stuff":

- Pick high-quality, durable equipment.
- Try it before you buy it.
- If you'll have to sit or stand on it, make sure the equipment is comfortable for you.
- Be certain it includes simple assembly instructions (if required).
- Look for an accompanying manual with instructions for use.
- Expect a reasonable warranty, easy maintenance, and available service if required.

Using It

Once you get your equipment home, remember these tips:

- Start slowly and gradually.
- Learn how to use it properly to minimize your risk of injury.
- Change your routine regularly to keep your activity interesting.
- Use a variety of equipment if you have more than one item.
- Read a book, listen to the radio, or watch TV while working out if your equipment and activity allow it (and you want to).

CHOOSING A CLASS OR FACILITY

Recreation centers, YWCAs and YMCAs, and fitness and health clubs offer a wide range of classes, facilities, and equipment. They also vary in philosophy and approach.

If you're thinking of signing up at a facility, it's important to find one that suits you. Visit at a time you would usually participate. Request a tour, or, if possible, just wander around and get a feel for the place. Talk to staff, to participants, and to friends who attend.

SIGN-UP CHECKLIST

Use the *Fitness Facility Checklist* to help you make a decision. There is no "passing grade," but the more checkmarks, the better the facility and the better your chances of safely sticking with your program.

FITNESS FACILITY CHECKLIST

Personal Issues

❑   Accessibility—it's close to home or work.

❑   Availability—operating hours are suitable.

❑   Attractiveness—the atmosphere feels comfortable and right.

Program Issues

❑   Facilities are clean and well ventilated.

❑   The flooring for exercise classes is made of shock-absorbing material.

❑   Equipment is well organized and in good working order.

❑   Appropriate preexercise screening is done. (The PAR-Q on p. 44 is a good example of this.)

❑   Attention is paid to exercise safety through proper instruction and appropriate class sizes.

❑   Participants are encouraged to go at their own paces.

❑   Education is provided through presentations, bulletin board material, handouts, and similar avenues.

❑   Staff take the time to get to know participants.

Professional Issues

❑   Staff are properly trained and certified by a recognized fitness organization.

❑   Costs or fees are reasonable for the services provided.

❑   Short-term or "try-us-out" memberships are available.

❑   The contract (if it's necessary to sign one) is fair, with the opportunity to cancel if you change your mind.

Once you've settled on a good facility, you may want to choose a specific class to attend—you can try Tai Chi, stretching, yoga, aerobics, and more. If you pick one, make sure it suits your *interests*. And match it up with your *aptitude*. Some classes offer a beginner-to-advanced progression. Others (many aerobics classes, for example) are labeled mild, moderate, or intense. Choose what's appropriate for you.

Home exercise routines, exercise classes, and individual training programs have their own special appeal. The structure and the noticeable progression and improvement can be both motivating and satisfying. The pure physical feeling of a "workout" is rewarding. After an invigorating session, you feel good—physically and psychologically. You feel as if you can take on the world!

PLAYING COURT SPORTS OR TEAM GAMES

Tell my older brother that it's time for a run and he'll yawn and go back to his newspaper. Tell him it's time for squash or a game of hockey, and he's heading out the door. Millions of others are like him.

Many things give games their special appeal, like competition, challenge, and camaraderie. Some sports take you outdoors, while all of them involve being active in the company of friends—the very essence of active living.

Sports and Games notes some popular activities you might consider. Following the list are a few tips to help you do them "right."

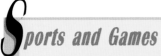
ports and Games

Court Sports		Team Games
Badminton*	Squash	Basketball
Handball	Tennis*	Hockey (floor and ice)
Racquetball		Soccer*
		Volleyball*

*These sports are not played exclusively indoors. When the weather's right, take them outside. As long as you're out there, why not try softball, touch football, or field hockey?

PLAY IT SAFE

Court sports and team games *are* lots of fun. But the fast action, stops and starts, confined space, and use of "tools and missiles"—rackets and sticks, balls and pucks—can lead to injuries and accidents.

Problems seem to occur most often with novices, the not-so-fit, "weekend" players, and older individuals taking up a sport for the first time. To avoid problems, it's important to play it safe. Here are a few suggestions:

- *Warm up.* Although many games players want to "get at it," a short warm-up is definitely in order to prepare you for the speed and demands of the game. Some easy running, or skating for those on ice, and a few stretches can do the trick. (The *Fast Five* in the *Stretch It* routine on pp. 67-70 will suffice.)

- *Get some instruction.* Whether it's swinging a tennis racket or kicking a soccer ball, poor technique is the cause of many injuries. If you're new to a sport or feel your skills could use some improvement, take lessons or get help from a more advanced player.

- *Wear proper footwear.* Stops, starts, and sideways movements require quality athletic footwear. Choose shoes that are right for you *and* for your sport.

- *Protect yourself.* Wearing proper protective equipment is essential. Needless (and often serious) eye injuries occur in squash and racquetball, for example, when players don't use protective eyewear. Whatever your sport, make sure you're outfitted properly. Look for protective gear that carries the seal of approval of a recognized safety association.

- *Stop on time.* Don't prolong games. Injuries often occur late in the action when fatigue builds.

- *Train for specific sports.* Joint injuries can occur because the surrounding muscles aren't strong enough to serve as good protectors. Performing sport-specific training routines should help avoid these injuries. Remember any injuries you do sustain might identify weaknesses and show the need for a corrective (and complementary) strength training program.

The fun, physical aspects of sports and games do much for your health and well-being. But if you're looking for fitness (particularly improvements in your stamina), be aware of your activity level. Take me and tennis, for example. I play it occasionally, poorly, and *strictly* for fun. Problem is, I spend more time hunting for the ball than I do hitting or chasing it. This might improve the stamina of my patience, but not my heart.

For fun *and* fitness, develop your skills, play against others of comparable fitness and skills, keep rest intervals to a minimum, and favor singles over doubles in any court sport you play.

CHAPTER

6

OUTDOORS

Four Favorites & More

*T*his chapter is a consumer's guide to a host of outdoor activities.

• **THE *FOUR FAVORITES*—**walking and hiking, running, cycling, and swimming*—invariably appear on the list of most popular activities in *any* survey of adult leisure-time activities. I've included swimming here because it has much in common with the other activities *and* because I hope you will pursue it outdoors whenever possible. Indoor swimming is fine, but river, lake, and ocean swimming offer special rewards.

• **THE *AND MORE*** part covers an A-to-Z list of outdoor endeavors. It's a long list—there's certainly something for everyone!

This chapter can't possibly present the nuances of all these activities. It does, however, provide what you need to get *started*. Basic how-to advice covers clothing and equipment, injury prevention and safety, and tips for starting and progressing. I've also tried to convey some of the feelings these activities bring to give you a sense for what they're all about. This may help you in making activity selections.

Three final thoughts before we move on:

- When purchasing any equipment or supplies for these outdoor activities, seek advice from *knowledgeable* sales staff at a *respected* equipment supply store.

- When pursuing these outdoor activities, remember that they generally improve your stamina. If *total* fitness is important to you, consider complementing these activities with a stretching routine and some strengthening exercises. See *Stretch It* (pp. 65-70) and *Strength Fit* (pp. 70-74) for more on this.

- Consider combining activities. This can bring a nice balance to your program and offer you variety and enjoyment. Any combination will do. Active living is the ultimate cross-training!

WALKING AND HIKING

 alking is easy. Easier, in fact, than standing on your head. As long as the same leg isn't used twice in succession, nothing much can go wrong.

Walking *is* a gentle activity. Set your own pace and you can walk comfortably with little risk of injury. It's so accessible, too. With a good pair of shoes and clothing to suit the weather, you can head out the door and get started.

THE FIRST STEPS

If brisk walking is for you, here are some things to remember.

- *Dress for the weather.* Wear layers of comfortable clothing that won't restrict movement. See pages 25-27 for clothing tips and advice.

- *Treat your feet.* Old "tennies" or loafers are just fine for the occasional stroll, but for regular brisk walking you'll want a good pair of shoes. (See *Shoe Enough* for help on this.)

Shoe Enough

Quality running shoes are great for walking. Look for these characteristics:

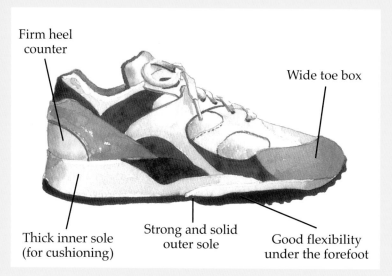

Firm heel counter

Wide toe box

Thick inner sole (for cushioning)

Strong and solid outer sole

Good flexibility under the forefoot

Shoes should be lightweight but sturdy and made of fabrics that allow the foot to breathe. New shoes should feel comfortable as soon as you put them on—not too wobbly, not too tight. Be sure to get a proper fit: Women may require a shoe that is narrower through the heel and in the arch. One last tip: Buy new shoes in the afternoon when your feet have "spread out" for the day.

- *Ease into it.* Start with short, easy walks (fifteen or twenty minutes or so) at least three times a week. Walk briskly when you're ready for it. Gradually extend the length of your walks, and go a little faster.

- *Do what comes naturally.* Your walking style should feel natural and right for you. Go for a stride length and a speed that are comfortable and smooth. If you like, swing your arms a little higher in front and back. Or bend them at the elbows and move them more vigorously (as is done in power walking and running).

- *Check the surface.* Be careful on ice and other slippery surfaces. When the weather is unfavorable (or too hot or cold), stride inside at a local mall, recreation center, or school.

- *Suit yourself.* Pick walking times that fit *your* routine and schedule.

WALK ON

You may find that your short daily outings lead to a desire for longer jaunts in the country. If so, get in touch with a hiking group in your area. (Staff at your local community center can probably tell you whom to contact.) Hiking groups welcome newcomers, so join in. It's a great way to explore new territory and make new friends.

While walking requires no special equipment (except good shoes as just noted), hiking is another matter. See *Boots and Packs* for more on these important items. Here are some other suggestions to make your hiking safe and pleasurable.

- *Be prepared.* When planning any hike, be ready for changes in the weather or a fall in the river! Pack rain gear, a change of clothes, and extra socks. Stock a small first-aid kit and take it along on every hike.

- *Fuel up.* Pack some food, then stop along the way for a light meal or energy snacks. Drink water at regular intervals to avoid dehydration. (Take a container of water with you if there won't be a good source available.)

- *Head for the hills.* Hiking often means covering some hilly terrain. For efficient effort, lean forward slightly and shorten your stride when going uphill. Traveling downhill may feel easy by comparison, but the legs work hard to cushion your weight on every step. Slow the pace and shorten your stride—your muscles will thank you afterward!

Boots and Packs

Choose boots and a pack that are comfortable and right for you. *Boots* come in three basic types:

Lightweight, low-cut boots

Heavier high-top boots

Heavy-duty, high-top, off-trail boots

Lightweight, low-cut boots are just fine for casual day hikes on modest terrain. Serious hiking calls for "serious" boots!

Packs also come in three basic varieties:

Fanny pack (the pouch sits across the lower back)

Day pack (small- to medium-sized backpack)

Larger pack (for "overnighters" and longer trips)

It's so easy to fit walking into your day. Walk to the store, to work, or to visit neighbors and you can cover a lot of ground. Leisurely outings with family or friends can offer you quiet times and special moments together.

I've certainly done my share of walking over the years. Nowadays, I especially enjoy Saturday morning walks with my Labrador retriever at my side and my two young sons romping on ahead. We circle through a big, rugged park up at the end of our road. The boys race through the trails, hide on one another, and play tag. I marvel at their energy and imagination, enjoy the sea breezes, and take in the view of distant islands and mountains. At times like this you can really slow down—and truly live for the moment.

"All walking is discovery," writes Hal Borland in *To Own the Streets and Fields*. "On foot we take the time to see things whole. We see trees as well as forests, people as well as crowds."

There's so much to enjoy on a simple, leisurely walk.

RUNNING

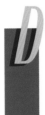

on't overdo it, underdo it

you aren't running because

you're in a hurry to get somewhere

—Fred Rohe, *The Zen of Running*

Running is a great activity, but it's not without its detractors. "Too demanding," some say. "Bad for the knees and the back," offer others. Take up running, they say, and you'll soon have problems. Professionals disagree. There is *nothing* unsafe about running itself. What's wrong is how some people pursue it. Pay close attention to the advice in this section and your running will be comfortable, safe, and enjoyable.

PREPARATION

Proper preparation means paying attention to surfaces, shoes, style, and safety.

- *Surfaces.* Roads and sidewalks *are* hard, but they're flat and predictable, and they present no problems if you wear good shoes. Trails and paths may take you through more interesting terrain, but you'll have to watch your footing. Loose gravel and dirt present risks of slipping, especially in rainy weather. (Ice brings the same risks in winter.) In these conditions, slow the pace and avoid bad spots.

- *Shoes.* Follow the *Shoe Enough* tips on page 85 when buying a new pair for running. With regular use, the soles will wear down, especially at the outside back corners (the natural landing spot). Keep an eye on this and replace your shoes when necessary.

- *Style.* See *Running Right* here for a few reminders. Get an experienced runner or a track coach to look at your style if you'd like some *personal* pointers. But don't complicate things. On the subject of style, famous Australian distance running coach Percy Cerutty once said, "Watch children run, and go and do likewise."

- *Safety.* Be wary of cars when crossing streets or if you run along a road. (If you must run on the shoulder, face the oncoming traffic.) Always cross with the lights or wait for a generous break in the traffic. If you run at night, wear bright clothing. (You might even consider reflective tape or a vest.) If you're concerned about running alone in certain places or after dark, find a partner. Run with someone compatible who also offers a measure of protection.

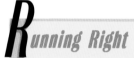

unning Right

Running with style means:

- a natural and comfortable stride length

- a soft heel or flat-foot landing

- a rock forward and gentle push off the toes

- an erect but relaxed posture, and

- bent arms that move forward and back (not sideways across the chest).

GETTING STARTED

There is no magic way to get into running. Following are two four-week beginner programs to consider. One I call the *Semiscientific Approach*, the other one the *Less Formal Approach*. Check them out, and try one if it seems as if it'll work for you. With either one, follow these guidelines:

- *Start with a short warm-up:* two or three minutes of easy (building to brisk) walking and the *Stretch It* routine (pp. 65-70; if time is tight, do at least the Fast Five.)

- *Go at a comfortable pace.* Use one of the pacing techniques described on page 90-91 if it will help you stay on track.
- *Move on.* Once you complete the program, add another day of running each week, or go a little farther each session.

Getting Started in Running—The Semiscientific Approach

Go at a pace that suits you. If it feels as if you're building up too quickly, repeat a week whenever you wish before going on to the next one.

Example: For Week 1, Day 1, you do fifteen seconds of running followed by forty-five seconds of walking. This one-minute sequence is repeated six times (that's the "× 6"), then followed by 1-1/2 minutes of walking. This brings you to 7-1/2 minutes. The whole sequence is then repeated, which brings you to fifteen minutes of total time.

WEEK 1	
	Day 1: (run 15 s + walk 45 s) × 6, walk 1-1/2 m; repeat
	Day 2: (run 20 s + walk 40 s) × 6, walk 1-1/2 m; repeat
	Day 3: (run 30 s + walk 30 s) × 6, walk 1-1/2 m; repeat

WEEK 2	
	Day 1: (run 40 s + walk 50 s) × 4, walk 1-1/2 m; repeat
	Day 2: (run 45 s + walk 45 s) × 4, walk 1-1/2 m; repeat
	Day 3: (run 50 s + walk 40 s) × 4, walk 1-1/2 m; repeat

WEEK 3	
	Day 1: (run 60 s + walk 60 s) × 3, walk 1-1/2 m; repeat
	Day 2: (run 75 s + walk 45 s) × 3, walk 1-1/2 m; repeat
	Day 3: (run 90 s + walk 60 s) × 2, walk 2-1/2 m; repeat

WEEK 4	
	Day 1: (run 1-1/2 m + walk 1 m) × 2, walk 2-1/2 m; repeat
	Day 2: (run 1-3/4 m + walk 1 m) × 2, walk 2 m; repeat
	Day 3: (run 2 m + walk 1-1/2 m) × 2, walk 1-1/2 m; (run 1-3/4 m + walk 1 m) × 2, walk 1 m

Key: s = seconds, m = minutes

After this, continue the gradual run/walk progression as it suits you.

Getting Started in Running— The Less Formal Approach

For those of you who don't like a "program," here's a different way to go:

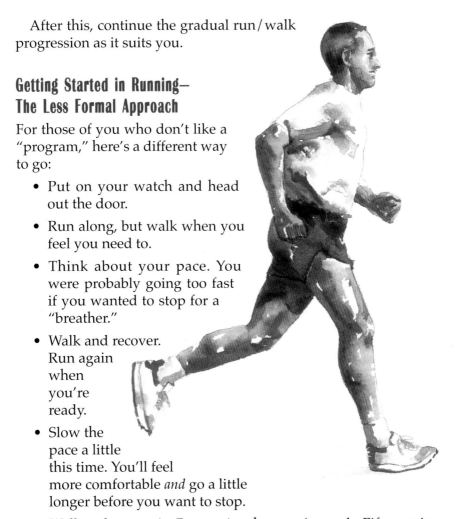

- Put on your watch and head out the door.

- Run along, but walk when you feel you need to.

- Think about your pace. You were probably going too fast if you wanted to stop for a "breather."

- Walk and recover. Run again when you're ready.

- Slow the pace a little this time. You'll feel more comfortable *and* go a little longer before you want to stop.

- Walk and rest again. Run again when you're ready. Fifteen minutes goes pretty quickly!

As time goes on you'll be running more and walking less. *Eventually* you'll be running fifteen minutes without stopping. This could be at the four-week mark, or a little before, or even long after. Everyone's different. Progress at your own rate!

INCREASING YOUR DISTANCE

One thing leads to the next. Get into running and you may soon find you want to go a little farther or enter a "fun run" or race. If so, here are some suggestions:

- *Make haste slowly.* As you add sessions to your program and distance to your runs, do it slowly and gradually. A general guideline is to increase your distance (or total running time) no more than 10% a week.

- *Find your optimum volume.* There's no use training to break three hours in the Boston Marathon if your body is happiest with a dozen miles a week at a nine-minute pace. Do what's right for you.

- *Seek training advice.* Training clinics and groups are available through many YMCAs and YWCAs, recreation centers, and local running clubs. See what's available in your community and consider getting involved. Along with the instruction, there's a chance to meet (and run with) others of a similar interest.

- *Keep things in perspective.* The more you run, the more time it takes away from other things. Training for 10K runs, marathons, and the like can be a real commitment—for the runners *and* all those close and important to them. Make sure there is family support for your efforts. Don't let your enthusiasm carry you away.

Running has come a long way since the boom of the 1970s. By the early 1980s, we had reached the height of fanaticism. We weren't hearing about the loneliness of the long-distance runner any more.

Running "grew up" during the 1980s. Fewer party conversations centered on features of running shoes, results of the latest race, or the pros and cons of carbohydrate loading.

In the 1990s we've settled down. There is less evangelism, but no less enthusiasm. The love affair with the marathon has become more rational. More runners really are "listening to their bodies," as the fitness specialists have been counseling all along.

There is a return to the simplicity of earlier years. For many people, running is simply one carefree step after another, returning when the time seems right, remembering not where or how far you ran, but only how good it felt along the way.

British Olympian Dave Bedford alluded to this in describing his own running: "I like to get out in the early morning when the sun's out. I get out in the park and take my vest off and I get a feeling of just moving smoothly in the sunlight."

This easy rhythm and sense of peace is there for *all* runners—elite athletes and fitness enthusiasts alike.

CYCLING

 e ought to replace the automobile with bicycles. . . . It would be better for our coronaries, our dispositions, and certainly our finances.

Dr. Irvine H. Page, one-time president of the American Heart Association, has been attributed with making this statement. He was on to something. While bicycling may not be a cure-all for our modern-day ills, it can do much to improve the quality of life for individuals *and* for the environment.

As a form of transportation, the bicycle is hard to beat. It's non-polluting and human-powered, and it takes up little space. The Worldwatch Institute goes so far as to herald the bicycle as "the vehicle for a small planet."

Beyond simple transportation, cycling can be a wonderful leisure-time activity for the whole family. Ride a little harder and it offers a workout that's tough to beat.

GET ROLLING

Whether you're into utility, leisure, or fitness riding, here are some things to remember.

- *Bike selection.* Mountain bikes are particularly popular, but there are also hybrids and road or racing bikes to choose from. If you're in the market for a new bicycle, pick one that suits both your pocketbook *and* your needs. The popular trend may not match your type of riding, so be sure to get a bike that is right for *you*.

- *Setup.* A good bicycle shop can make sure that your choice is the right size and can adjust handlebars, seat, and other parts so it's comfortable for you. Seat placement is particularly important. Make sure the seat is horizontal (to minimize stress on the lower back) and set at a height that allows a slight bend in the knee when your leg is extended.

- *Style.* Sit so your weight is evenly distributed over the seat, handlebars, and pedals. Pedal at a comfortable and steady speed, changing gears to adjust to hills, wind conditions, and your level of fitness (and fatigue).

- *Starting.* If you're a real beginner, take it easy! Avoid big hills at first. Don't venture off to work or school until you're ready for it. Severe breathlessness or tired and sore legs means you're building up too quickly. Three or four rides a week—fifteen or twenty minutes each time—are enough to begin.

- *Safety.* Donald Pruden has covered the key safety points in *Around Town Cycling:* Be aware. Be defensive. Be predictable. Be visible. Night riding calls for lights, reflectors, and bright clothing. Remember that road and traffic regulations apply to bicycles, too. And *always* wear a helmet! Look for one with a seal of approval from your national safety association. The helmet should have a hard shell and a foam liner and offer a snug and comfortable fit.

Case for the Helmet

For: Head injuries account for about 85% of bicycle accident fatalities. Wearing a helmet decreases the risk of a head injury in a crash by nearly 80%.

Against: The only arguments against wearing a helmet are that they're not comfortable and they're not "cool" (as in unbecoming, not the opposite of hot).

The verdict: Well worth wearing! There is *no* trouble in finding a helmet that's comfortable. And how much better to be uncool and alive than the opposite!

MOVING ON

Beyond fun rides with the family and short trips to the grocery store, the bicycle is a many-splendored vehicle. It's great for commuting, fitness riding, *and* touring. With comfortable clothing and cycling shoes and gloves, you're ready for action.

- *Commuting.* In addition to providing health benefits, cycle commuting saves gas, parking costs, and wear and tear on your car. If you have a considerable distance to travel, you could get a bike rack for the car and do a drive–ride combination. Look for quieter, safer streets and byways if traffic is a concern. The bicycle offers big environmental benefits, especially when replacing short automobile trips. (These create the most pollution because a cold engine does not fire efficiently.) Given that most commuting trips are short (half in North America are less than five miles), the bicycle is an important part of effective clean-air strategies.

- *Fitness riding.* If you get into riding for fitness, there is no way to increase your distance other than slowly, gradually, patiently. In cycling as in other sports, there are all sorts of sophisticated training plans to help you improve. But as you progress, don't lose sight of the simplicity and freedom of the ride. Remember the words of Eddie Merckx, Belgian cyclist and many-time winner of the Tour de France. When asked the secret to success, he said, "Ride lots." If you want to ride lots in the company of others, inquire at your local bike shop about cycling clubs and groups in your area. The enthusiasm and energy of the group can add much to your riding experience.

- *Touring.* If you move on to touring, ease into it. A veteran cyclist friend of mine warns, "For heaven's sake, don't go and try to ride a thirty-five-mile day right away. Start with five miles for a while, then ten, and so on. . . . It could be months and months before you're ready for the longer rides." Your legs need to grow "cycling fit," and you have to get used to sitting on the bike seat for longer and longer periods. Take it a step at a time. Enjoy the outing and the day.

Spring Tune-Up Checklist

☐ *Tires*—in good condition and properly inflated

☐ *Wheels*—in true, no broken spokes, clean rims

☐ *Brakes*—operational and providing sufficient braking power

☐ *Drive train*—properly lubricated, adjusted, clean, in good working order

☐ *Handlebars**—set correctly in relation to the seat

☐ *Seat**—horizontal and at the correct height

☐ *Bearing sets* (headset, bottom bracket, axles, pedals)—properly lubed and adjusted

An annual safety and road-readiness check of your bicycle by specialists at your local shop makes good sense. Should you want to do minor repairs and maintenance yourself, check out courses available through schools, community colleges, and some bike shops.

*The positioning of the seat and handlebars in relation to one another will depend on your type of bike, handlebar style, your height, and other comfort factors.

As I write this, my trusty twenty-year-old, ten-speed bicycle is resting and rusting in the carport. It has served me well in years of cycle commuting, bouts of fitness riding, and occasional, casual touring. These days it is called into action for short rides to soccer practice with my sons and for weekend outings where we enjoy sights and smells and I try to instill in the boys the rules of the road and the importance of bicycle safety.

I'm thankful for my earlier fitness riding and touring. It helps me to fully appreciate what others say about the activity. If you get into regular cycling, you may truly come to understand what Sue Browder meant in the *American Biking Atlas and Touring Guide*: "Biking . . . invigorates and brings you in touch with what's happening around you and in tune with nature. Experience the romantic changes of the day—a crisp dawn, a sunny noon, a starry night. Feel the breezes, taste the salt spray off the ocean, touch a redwood. Enjoy the best things about being alive."

Others have said much the same. At a time when many seem to be in a hurry to get somewhere, cyclists of all people know that fastest is not necessarily best.

SWIMMING

 wimming is one activity you can enjoy lying down.

Water has a dual personality. Its buoyancy and support act as a cushion allowing graceful and gentle movement. But move with greater force and the water resists. It's a pleasant and helpful contradiction.

The water has something for everyone. It's ideal for those with back problems, arthritis, and other joint disorders. Water exercise programs are popular with older adults—the buoyancy and support soften the infirmities of advancing age.

For fitness, along with improved stamina, swimming brings a balanced development—upper and lower body strength and suppleness—that few activities can match. For fun, there are all sorts of opportunities—synchronized swimming, skin and scuba diving, water polo (for the skillful), and inner-tube water polo (for the playful).

GET WET

If a swim-to-fitness program is for you, here are some things to think about.

- *Suits.* Quick-drying nylon–lycra blends are the choice of novice and champion alike. A swim coach I know estimates about eight months' use from a suit (at 1-1/2 hours a day in the water). This works out to a few cents a session.

- *Goggles.* Goggles improve vision, offer comfort, and help reduce or eliminate irritation and itchiness that can result from exposure to chemically treated pool water. If your eyes trouble you after swimming, consider adding goggles to your equipment list. (If you wear contacts and want to wear them when you swim, get tight-fitting goggles and always clean your contacts immediately after swimming. Prescription goggles are available as an alternative.)

- *Ear plugs.* Public health codes ensure properly maintained pools, so ear infections from swimming aren't that common. Nevertheless, if you're susceptible to the problem, ear plugs are a wise precaution.

- *Lessons.* If you are a poor swimmer or have never learned to swim, lessons are a good investment and a logical starting point. When you master the basic strokes, you double your returns. Each session in the water will bring improved skills *and* fitness. They build on one another.

- *Water exercise.* Whether the class is called swimnastics, aquarobics, or swim and trim, participants are doing exercises in the water. Try a class if you think it might appeal to you, or add some in-the-water bending, stretching, and strengthening exercises to your swimming routine. If you aren't a proficient swimmer, then walking, running, skipping, hopping, bounding, and paddling are all great ways to be active in the water while your skills and fitness improve.

STROKE ON

Here are a few more tips to keep you in the swim:

- *Swim/rest.* The same advice holds here as for other activities in this chapter: Start with fifteen to twenty minutes of moving several times a week. Continuous swimming should be your eventual goal, but if you're new to the activity follow the "swim/rest" principle. Swim a length (or two) and rest when you need it. Walk around or do some flutter kicking or gentle water exercise until you're ready to go again.

- *Pace yourself.* If you're using pulse counting to monitor the intensity of your program, lower your target rate by two beats in the ten-second count. (For reasons that physiologists don't fully understand, we tend to have a lower maximum heart rate when swimming than when running, for example.) Use the Heart Rate Target Zone chart on page 48 as a starting point, then adjust your targets downward. This lower rate will help prevent overexertion.

- *Go for variety.* Sidestroke, breaststroke, and elementary backstroke are the easy half of swimming's six strokes. Their glide phase gives them their "resting stroke" label. The front crawl, back crawl, and butterfly require more strength and endurance. Mix resting strokes with the strenuous ones to keep moving *and* to keep things interesting.

*W**ater Safety*

Be safe. Follow this simple advice:

- Never swim alone. Use the "buddy system," even in a pool.

- Take special precautions when swimming in a river, a lake, or the ocean. Don't overestimate your abilities *or* underestimate distances.

- Take extreme care in or near the water with infants and young children who can't yet swim. Be an attentive *lifeguard*.

For more information on water safety, contact the Red Cross office nearest you.

The quiet and the motion are two of the special things about swimming. Walking, running, and cycling let you attune to your surroundings and flow with its changing personality. If you swim in a pool you don't experience these daily differences, so in time you come to focus on the peace, the quiet, and the movement.

Lake or ocean swimming adds to the experience. Years ago, when running was the focus of my physical activity, I remember visiting a friend at his lakeside cottage. My "swimmer" friend said to "runner" me, "It's *not* like a pool. *Every* day is different." He was right. Wind and waves made for distant bobbing islands as we edged toward the neighbor's dock. Sun and clouds brought hues of blue and green to our water.

Water, indeed, buoys the body. The action of swimming is graceful, relaxing, and pleasing. Even more, you find that the moving, the wind, the waves, and those distant bobbing islands buoy the spirit.

MORE OUTDOOR ACTIVITIES

ature is willing to give us nearly everything we could wish for, providing we take it from her in exactly the way she wants us to.

The *choices* we make in our leisure-time activities affect us in many ways. The activities on the following list are all *human-powered*. (Well, almost all—one involves a horse and another needs the wind.) Like the "four favorites" discussed in earlier sections of the chapter, these activities offer personal health benefits. And done in a careful and caring manner, they need not have a detrimental effect on the environment.

Unfortunately, the same cannot be said for *non–human-powered* activities. Activities using motorized recreational vehicles, like powerboats, snowmobiles, and all-terrain vehicles (ATVs), require less physical activity. And by their very nature they can be damaging to the environment *whenever* they are done.

This book cannot do justice to all of the outdoor opportunities available, but I can at least encourage you to make wise choices. The A-to-Z list offers a wealth of activities to consider. Some require snow; others need warm weather and water. Some, like mountaineering, may mean a little travel. Others you can do in your own backyard.

Outdoor Active Living Choices: A to Z

Why not try . . .

Archery	Kayaking
Bocci ball	Mountaineering
Canoeing	Orienteering
Cross-country skiing	Rowing
Downhill skiing	Sailboarding
Fishing	Sailing
Gardening	Shuffleboard
Golfing	Skateboarding
Hang gliding	Snorkeling/scuba diving
Horseback riding	Snowboarding
Ice-skating	Snowshoeing
In-line (or roller) skating	Tobogganing/sledding

I'm sure the list is bigger. Anybody know of an activity that begins with X?

OUTDOOR ACTIVITY GUIDE

Here are a few suggestions for fun and safety when participating.

- *Consider your options.* If improving your fitness is part of your reason for participating, choose your activities accordingly. Skating is more demanding than shuffleboard, for example, and canoeing tops sailing (into *or* with the wind!).

- *Outfit yourself properly.* Your activities will dictate your equipment needs. Comfort is crucial in anything you wear. Special protective gear is essential for some activities (wrist guards, elbow and knee pads, and a helmet for in-line skating, for example), while accessories like a pack are necessary for others. A first-aid kit (and food and water) should be on your list of supplies for hiking, cross-country skiing, and the like.

- *Be weather-wise.* Tips for participating in hot and cold weather appear in the *Taking Care* section of chapter 2. Suggestions to help you dress for the occasion are also included there.

- *Chart your course.* Some activities take you off the beaten track. If so, a map and compass can be lifesavers. Topographical maps may be obtained from your local parks department or forest service; compasses are available at recreational equipment stores. Take a course or get a guidebook so you'll know how to use them properly.

Much has been written about the "outdoor experience." Colin Fletcher, an author and a hiking enthusiast, describes it as well as anyone. He has written of mountains, snow country, and other places. About the desert he says, "You rediscover, every time you go back, the cleanness that exists in spite of the dust, the complexity that underlies the apparent openness, and the intricate web of life that stretches over the apparent barrenness; but above all you rediscover the echoing silence that you had thought you would never forget."

Urban living in the electronic age makes it far too easy to forget what's around us. But if you get outdoors—and off the beaten track—in a human-powered activity, you can reconnect with nature. When you do, you are reminded of its rhythm and beauty, and of our place in the overall scheme of things.

CHAPTER 7

COMPLETING THE PICTURE

Other Healthy Habits

hen you embrace active living, you *take up* something. Physical activity is what you take up, and if you add the *right* activities to your daily routine they can be positive and pleasurable from the beginning.

Not so with other things. If you want to improve your eating habits, lose weight, stop smoking, or drink less alcohol, for example, you have to *give up* something. This can be challenging, difficult, even not much fun.

This chapter addresses these other things to complete the picture of health:

- *TAKING STOCK* (assessing your status)
- *EATING RIGHT* (nutrition)
- *STAYING COOL* (stress management)
- *BREAKING FREE* (smoking)
- *STAYING REAL* (alcohol and drugs)

Along with a short discussion in each topic area are some tips for taking charge. The final section—*Being Happy*—covers some other less tangible but nonetheless important issues.

If *you'd* like to nurture some new, more healthful habits, start by completing the action plan in the first section of the chapter. Then, as you progress, keep Mark Twain's wise advice in mind. "Habit is habit," he said, "not to be flung out the window by anyone, but coaxed downstairs a step at a time." Start winning in one area, then move on to the next. A series of small successes add up to one big victory.

TAKING STOCK

If you'd like to make some lifestyle changes, take a few minutes to complete the *Health Habits Action Plan*. Peruse the *Tips for Taking Charge* throughout the chapter to guide you in your planning. Refer to your plan from time to time to remind you of your thoughts and desires and to check on how you're doing.

HEALTH HABITS ACTION PLAN

I would like to make changes in the following area(s):

☐ Diet and nutrition   ☐ Smoking

☐ Body weight   ☐ Alcohol and other drugs

☐ Stress management

These are the changes I would like to make:

Here are some things that will help me to succeed:

This is *what I will do* to get started:

EATING RIGHT

've been on a diet for two weeks and all I've lost is two weeks.

—Totie Fields

When choosing foods to enhance your well-being, strive for a diet that is varied, balanced, and moderate.

• *Variety* means a wide selection among the four food groups *and* within each group. As much as possible, choose foods close to their natural state, like fresh fruits and vegetables when they're in season.

• *Balance* refers to both nutrients and calories. To ensure a balance of nutrients follow the *Good Eating Guide*. A balance of calories comes from an appropriate number of calories consumed in food and expended through physical activity. A proper balance will help lead to a *healthy* weight.

• *Moderation* means being modest in your serving sizes and limiting your intake of fat, alcohol, caffeine, salt, and sugar. By being moderate, you can avoid eating too much or too often or making food choices that are too limited.

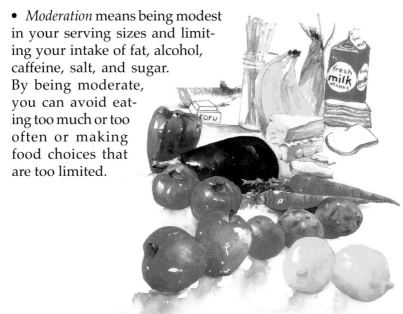

Good Eating Guide*

For a balanced, varied diet, consume a range of foods from the four groups as shown.

Grain products—5-12 servings each day

Examples of one serving: 1 slice of bread; 3/4 cup of cooked cereal or 30 grams of ready-to-eat cereal; 1/2 cup of cooked rice or pasta; half a bun, bagel, or pita.

Vegetables and fruit—5-10 servings each day

Examples of one serving: 1/2 cup of vegetables, fruit, or juice; 1 medium potato, carrot, peach, banana (etc.); 1 cup of salad. (Try for at least 2 servings of vegetables.)

Milk products—*2-3 servings each day for children 4-9 years; 3-4 servings for youths 10-16; 2-4 servings for adults; and 3-4 servings for pregnant and breast-feeding women*

Examples of one serving: 1 cup of milk; 3/4 cup of yogurt; 50 grams of hard cheese; 2 slices of processed cheese.

Meat and alternatives—2-3 servings

Examples of one serving: 50 to 100 grams (the size of a deck of cards) of meat, poultry, or fish; 1/2 to 1 cup of cooked beans; 1-2 eggs; 1/3 cup of tofu; 2 tbsp of peanut butter.

*Based on *Canada's Food Guide to Healthy Eating*, 1992.

TIPS FOR TAKING CHARGE

Here are some suggestions to keep your eating on track:

- *Watch your fat intake.* Choose skim, 1%, or 2% milk and lower fat cheeses. Choose lean meat, fish, and poultry, trim off visible fat, and avoid coatings and frying. Use meat alternatives like tofu, dried peas, beans, or lentils more often.

- *Check your calcium.* Regular physical activity will help keep your bones healthy and strong, but adequate calcium in the diet is essential, too. Milk products and fish (especially sardines, herring, mackerel, and canned salmon—all with the bones) are particularly good sources of calcium.

- *Watch your iron.* Active people must be sure to get enough iron in their diets. Excellent sources include liver, dark meat, baked beans, dried fruit, and dark green leafy vegetables. Absorption of iron from plant sources can be enhanced when accompanied by some vitamin C in the meal.

- *Eat a hearty breakfast.* With a nutritious breakfast under your belt, you'll concentrate better, you'll be less likely to suffer from hunger headaches, and you won't be tempted to overeat during the day. Breakfast should provide a quarter to a third of your daily requirements for energy and nutrients.

- *Get the water habit.* Drink *lots* of water! Juice and milk are great fluids, too. On the other hand, you should limit your intake of coffee, tea, cocoa, cola, and alcohol. They stimulate the body to excrete more fluids and can lead to dehydration (a common cause of fatigue).

- *Adopt new eating styles with care.* If you're thinking of going vegetarian, for example, see a registered dietitian for advice, suggested reading, and good cookbooks.

Thin Is Not In

The "thin is in" image portrayed by advertisers and the media can lead to inappropriate dieting and unhealthy underweight. What you should be striving for is a *healthy* weight—not thinness. To do this:

Avoid extremes. Don't drastically reduce calories, eliminate essential foods, or exercise endlessly.

Focus on active living. Pursue activities you enjoy and participate with friends.

Be realistic. We weren't all meant to be the same size and shape, so don't impose fantasy standards of slimness on yourself. Aim for a *healthy* weight for *you*.

Make eating a pleasurable experience. Slow down and enjoy the aroma and taste of food. Whenever possible, make meals a time for companionship, talking, and laughter.

Treat yourself, too! Active people can enjoy a few extra foods—sweets and treats—from time to time. The key, of course, is moderation.

STAYING COOL

 or peace of mind, resign as general manager of the universe.

—Larry Eisenberg

The amount of stress you face—and how you handle it—is another lifestyle factor that greatly affects your health.

Although stress has a bad reputation, a certain amount of it is essential to well-being. Some types of stress are actually good for us. Anticipation of a positive event, excitement, and extreme happiness are positive "stressors." Fear, anger, and guilt, on the other hand, are negative ones.

Regardless of the nature of the stressor, the body responds to it with a number of physiological changes. More adrenaline is released into the bloodstream, muscles tense, breathing quickens, and heart rate and blood pressure rise. This reaction, known as the "fight or flight" response, was important in primitive times when movement was crucial to survival. People did, in fact, fight or flee.

This innate physiological response to stress is still with us, but now we are more often denied the opportunity of "putting 'em up" or taking off. Repeated stress, if unresolved, can lead to serious problems.

Early signs of unresolved stress include sleeplessness, headaches, irritability, depression, and fatigue. Poorly managed over a long period, stress can lead to health problems such as permanent high blood pressure, colitis, ulcers, and heart disease.

The key to preventing problems is not to avoid stress entirely (which isn't possible anyway) but to harness it and know your limits. This means identifying the *negative* stressors in your life and learning how to cope with them effectively.

*T*he Exercise Connection

Regular physical activity is an effective antidote to stress. Dr. Hans Selye, world renowned for his stress research, described it as setting up a "cross-resistance" against emotional stress. Dr. William D. Ross put it nicely in *Life and Health* when he wrote, "Deliberate and appropriate exercise enables modern man to release psychological tension and achieve physical relaxation."

TIPS FOR TAKING CHARGE

There are many ways to help deal with stress. Here are a few ideas:

- *Balance work and recreation.* Long hours of work, even when it's work you enjoy, eventually take their toll. Enjoyable leisure-time pursuits help restore energy and enthusiasm. Recreational activities can also provide satisfaction and fulfillment to balance other areas of your life where you may feel frustrated or where you haven't enough control.

- *Accept what you can't change.* Try not to get upset about circumstances that are beyond your control. Find areas in your life where you can exercise control, then act effectively to reach your goals.

- *Avoid hassles.* Hassles like traffic jams and lineups at the supermarket can be irritating, so do your best to avoid them. If you can't, then try to adapt. Smile and listen to the radio in slow-moving traffic. Talk to others in the checkout line. Develop a more relaxed attitude toward daily chores.

- *Set priorities; don't rush.* You can be active and busy without being hurried. At work and at home, determine priorities, then strive to accomplish things in both a logical fashion and a reasonable length of time.

- *Keep a diary.* Stress can come from not being sure what you want. A diary is a wonderful tool for self-discovery; when you record your emotions and experiences—the good as well as the bad— you can start to see important patterns emerge. You needn't write in your diary every day, but you need to reread it regularly.

- *Talk to others.* Problems can seem worse when you keep them to yourself. Make adequate time to deepen friendships, and share your concerns with a trusted friend or relative. This can help you see your situation in a new light, which may be the first step toward a constructive solution. If your problems seem to be getting out of hand, don't hesitate to seek professional counseling.

- *Learn to relax.* Some people choose biofeedback, meditation, or relaxation techniques to help manage stress. Why not explore these possibilities? Take a little time each day to put your feet up, close your eyes, slow your breathing, and think about pleasant things. A short daily "time-out" helps you feel refreshed.

- *Listen to your body.* It will tell you when you're pushing too hard. When warning signs like sleeplessness or fatigue appear, slow down. Have fun! Indulge yourself. Enjoy life's little pleasures.

A final important part of stress management is simply *knowing yourself*—and acting accordingly. If you thrive on a busy (but not too busy!) schedule, then pursue it. If you're happier living more leisurely, you should do it. Discover the lifestyle that best suits you, then live it. To do otherwise—to go against your nature—would be stressful.

BREAKING FREE

 t makes absolutely no sense to put something in your mouth and set it on fire.

—Dr. George Sheehan

Cigarette smoking is the single biggest cause of preventable premature death in the developed world. It is a significant factor in disability and death due to lung cancer, heart disease, emphysema, and chronic bronchitis. But you probably know this already.

Here are some lesser known facts: about 20% of fires and more than 40% of all fire deaths are smoking related. Children whose parents smoke are much more likely to smoke than those whose parents do not.

What about "secondhand smoke"? Sidestream smoke—that emitted by the burning tip of a cigarette, cigar, or pipe—contains higher concentrations of many cancer-producing chemicals than does inhaled smoke. This evidence has led municipalities to pass bylaws regarding smoke-free public places, companies to develop workplace smoking policies, and airlines to provide smoke-free travel.

Successful smoking cessation depends on a number of factors, including the duration and intensity of the smoking habit; the smoker's age, sex, and personal stress levels; and the support and encouragement of family, co-workers, and friends. Kicking the habit *isn't* easy, but anyone *can* do it.

Great Gains

If you're a smoker wanting to quit, you'll have much to gain from doing so:

You'll feel better.

You'll have more energy.

Your senses of taste and smell will improve.

Your risk of all smoking-related diseases will be greatly reduced.

You'll save money.

You'll contribute to a more healthful environment for everyone around you.

TIPS FOR TAKING CHARGE

If you're a smoker and you've decided it's time to quit, there are three time-proven steps in the process: getting ready, quitting, and staying free.

- *Getting ready to quit.* Start by analyzing your smoking habits. Determine what situations and feelings make you want to smoke. If you know and recognize these, you can devise ways to cope with them once you've stopped. Determine any barriers to quitting (fear of failure, the prospect of weight gain, the loss of something you enjoy, etc.), so you can deal with these as well. Then list your benefits in quitting, set a quit date, and decide on your rewards for success. Seek support from family and friends (this is very important!), and make a contract with yourself if you think it will help.

- *Quitting.* When your quit date comes, you can either taper off or go "cold turkey." (Both methods have their advantages, so you must choose the one that suits you.) Be ready to deal with some possible effects of nicotine withdrawal, like irritability, increased appetite, fatigue, and insomnia. Physical activity can be an effective antidote to these potential problems. It can have a positive effect on your mood, burn calories and help control your weight, give you extra energy, and help you relax and sleep better. See your doctor for other ways to deal with nicotine withdrawal if it proves to be troublesome for you.

- *Staying free.* Successful coping strategies include talking to your supporters, deep breathing, avoiding temptation (recall your list of things that trigger your desire to smoke), and, of course, getting more physical activity. Try low-calorie snacks, gum, toothpicks, or carrot sticks as substitutes for cigarettes. If you resume smoking, don't consider yourself a failure. Many people require several tries before they kick the habit for good. Get set, and try again!

- *Use community helpers.* Though self-motivation is the key to smoking cessation and most people "go it alone," there are a variety of groups, programs, and community resources available to assist those who wish to quit. Contact your local cancer society office or talk to your doctor if you feel you need some help.

There are things we *all* can do to help create a smoke-free environment for everyone. We can support *anyone* trying to quit by being nonjudgmental and recognizing how difficult a task it can be. (It's not just a case of willpower.) We can (politely!) request that smokers who are not complying with smoking restrictions in designated areas do so for the health and comfort of others. We can encourage employers to provide a smoke-free workplace. And we can support community efforts to eliminate smoking from public places.

Finally, by *not* smoking, we set a good example for all young people who—for the health of it—deserve to be smoke-free for life.

STAYING REAL

hen patterns are broken, new worlds can emerge.

—Tuli Kupferberg

Scientists define a drug as any substance, other than food, that is taken to change the way the body or mind functions. The two main classes of drugs are prescription and nonprescription (or over-the-counter), both of which are obtained at pharmacies. (Many over-the-counter medications may also be obtained at nonpharmacy outlets.)

Then there are social drugs. The alcohol in wine, beer, and spirits, the nicotine in tobacco, and the caffeine in coffee, tea, cocoa, and cola drinks are all "social drugs." These are sometimes called "invisible drugs" because many people are unaware that they are, in fact, drugs.

The final category is the one casually referred to as "street drugs." This group includes illicit drugs like amphetamines (speed), LSD, cocaine (and its derivative, crack), heroin, and marijuana and hashish.

PRESCRIPTION AND OVER-THE-COUNTER DRUGS

These must be taken as directed *and* with care to obtain the desired effect. If you experience any unpleasant side effects or reactions, you should get in touch with your physician or pharmacist immediately.

Alcohol can interact with drugs as well, so, as a general rule, don't drink alcohol when you are on any medication—prescription *or* over-the-counter—unless your doctor and pharmacist approve.

As much as possible, use a single pharmacy to ensure a complete and up-to-date record of your medications.

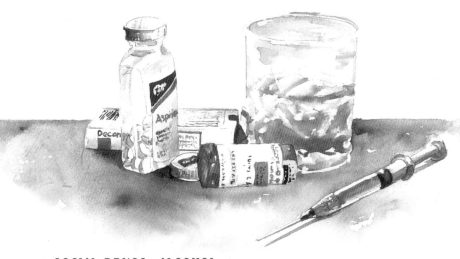

SOCIAL DRUGS—ALCOHOL

Drinking alcohol in moderation shouldn't be a problem, but if you consume several drinks a day or you go on occasional binges, you risk real physical harm. Excessive drinking can cause ulcers, liver damage, neurological disorders, cancer (of the mouth, larynx, and esophagus), and malnutrition (alcohol can fill you up but its calories have few or no nutrients). Immoderate drinking can lead to alcoholism, a disease whose effects harm not only alcoholics but also those who dearly love them.

If you drink moderately, you may never face any of these concerns. Nevertheless, it does pay to have a healthy regard for the potential problems associated with alcohol.

STREET (AND SPORTS) DRUGS

Street drugs are illegal, potentially addicting, and extremely hazardous to health. An additional risk is the unknown—they are not always what the sellers allege them to be. For drugs in this category, health professionals say, quite simply, "To use them is to abuse them."

Any use of drugs to enhance physical performance or physique is also drug abuse. We hear all too often of amphetamines and anabolic steroids being used in professional sport and, sadly, even among college and high school athletes. Such drug use has no place in sport, where fair play is valued, *or* in a healthy approach to life.

TIPS FOR TAKING CHARGE

Following are a few suggestions relating to drug use and abuse:

- *Use drugs wisely.* Prescription and over-the-counter drugs are designed to do certain things and to be taken for specified periods. Sleeping medications, for example, can be helpful for short-term relief, but they lose their effectiveness after a few weeks. Dependence on these medications can occur quite quickly, and adverse health effects can result from long-term use. Drug therapies should therefore be reevaluated regularly. (See *Sleep Tight* for nondrug ways to deal with sleeplessness.)

- *Follow directions.* When taking prescription and over-the-counter drugs, carefully follow the prescription therapy or the directions for use as discussed earlier. If you have any questions about dosage, possible side effects, or interactions with other drugs, talk to your pharmacist or physician.

- *Drink moderately or not at all.* If you have any concerns about your own drinking habits or those of someone close to you—a family member, friend, or co-worker—deal with them. Seek professional help if necessary.

- *Stay real.* If you suspect that someone close to you is taking street drugs, address the problem without delay. Get proper medical care immediately. (*Watch Out for the Ones You Love* offers some warning signs to look for.)

- *Drive safely.* Drinking, drugs, and driving do *not* mix. It's a common message these days, but it's important enough to bear repeating. Alcohol impairs the ability to judge speed, time, and distance and is a major cause of traffic accidents and deaths. Medications containing depressants can cause impairments similar to those brought on by alcohol. Any drugs in combination can produce a synergistic—more than "1 + 1"—effect. One drink and a dose of cough medicine or decongestant, for example, can quadruple the drug effects and the driving impairment.

"Stay real" is the wise advice Health Canada gives in an educational booklet about marijuana and hashish. It is particularly important advice for these substances, but it's an appropriate caution when someone is considering the use of *any* mood-altering drug.

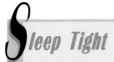

Sleep Tight

If you have *persistent* difficulty in sleeping and medical problems have been ruled out as the cause, there are drug-free ways to help you get a good night's sleep. Try the following for six weeks. They are simple habits, but they can have a long-lasting effect.

- Establish a consistent routine. Get up at the same time every day, using an alarm clock if needed.
- Avoid napping, especially later in the day.
- Avoid coffee, tea, and other beverages containing the stimulant caffeine after dinnertime. Smokers should refrain from smoking in the evening.
- Avoid heavy meals and alcohol close to bedtime. A light carbohydrate snack before bed is fine and may even help promote sleep.
- Create an atmosphere conducive to sleep. Keep the room at a comfortable temperature, and control the light and noise.
- Don't go to bed until you are drowsy. Once in bed, relax and think pleasant thoughts to help you drift off to sleep.

Watch Out for the Ones You Love

Here are some warning signs of illicit drug use. If a family member or friend is exhibiting these behaviors, you should take immediate action to explore the problem.

- Abrupt change in mood or attitude
- Sudden decline in attendance or performance at school, at work, or in other activities
- Unusual temper flare-ups
- Impaired relationship with family and friends
- Increased borrowing of money
- Heightened secrecy about actions and possessions
- Associating with a new group of friends

BEING HAPPY

 man is as happy as his mind allows him to be.

—Abraham Lincoln

This whole book is about healthy habits. Most of it covers the active living part, a great starting point for anyone looking for improved personal health. Previous sections in this chapter considered lifestyle habits that add to our picture of health.

This is all pretty tangible stuff. Make some changes—a little more of this, a little less of that—and improved health will surely follow. But there are other, less tangible things that are just as important.

Mental health, emotional well-being, and *spiritual wellness* are just a few of the terms used to cover this side of it. While my term may make it sound simpler than it really is, I've chosen to cover these aspects of health under the "happiness" umbrella.

Health and happiness are definitely related. And they build on one another. Happiness can come from the simple pleasure of enjoying physical activity. And it can come, in turn, from the "good feeling" that good health brings.

But happiness also comes from a sense of contentment, a sense of belonging, and a sense of purpose. These characteristics relate to *attitude* and *involvement*.

Although a certain amount of solitude is healthy, research shows the importance of being involved, or "plugged in." Extreme isolation and lack of social support can lead to ill health, whereas active community involvement and a network of friends contribute to positive health.

Involvement can come in many forms. It might be coaching your daughter's soccer team or helping organize a community clean-up campaign. It might be joining a group, taking a class, attending a public lecture, or enjoying a concert. It means cultivating friendships and having at least one close friend in whom you can confide.

Attitude is the other part of it. We all know and are inspired by people with a "no worries" approach to life. These people, no matter their circumstances, have a certain hardiness. They go through life with a sense of hopefulness and optimism, generally seeing the brighter side, the lighter side. They enjoy today, not dwelling on the past that can't be changed or fretting about things in the future over which they have no control.

This special attitude also involves an openness—to new people, new ideas, and new experiences, and to planning, setting goals, and looking forward to new challenges. The late, great baseball pitcher Satchel Paige captured this attitude to life (in his own special way) in his now famous Rules for Living. In Rule #6 he said, "Don't look back, something may be gaining on you."

*A*ctivity Works

People who pursue regular physical activity say their sessions leave them relaxed, refreshed, and more energetic. Research also shows that activity has a positive effect on mood. Short bouts of activity lead to significant, temporary decreases in tension, depression, and anxiety.

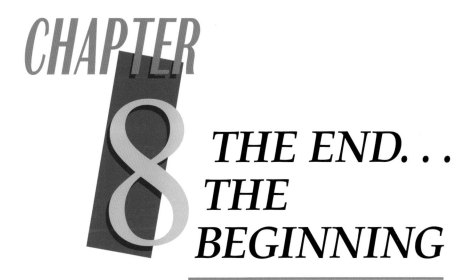

CHAPTER 8

THE END. . . THE BEGINNING

> *We act as though comfort and luxury were the chief requirements of life, when all we really need to make us happy is something to be enthusiastic about.*
>
> —Charles Kingsley

Well, it's just about the end for me. I've done my part, done all that I can do. And now, perhaps, comes a beginning for you.

Your *beginning* might mean including just a little more activity in your daily routine. Or it could mean heading out to the park with the kids more often. Or cycle commuting to work. Or trying a new activity that you've always wanted to do but somehow never have found the time for.

This book has been largely about beginning—about developing healthy habits, adopting an active way of life. To this end, I have provided all sorts of information and advice, and it was not too difficult really. It's all so straightforward and tangible.

But along with the advice, I have tried for something more. I've tried to convey some of the deeper, more meaningful aspects of active living. In chapter 4 I talked of the 3 Ss of fitness. Perhaps what I'm getting at in this chapter could be called the 3 Ss of active living:

---

the Spirit of it,
its Sense of place,
and its gentle Simplicity.

I've called on the words of others along the way to help capture the *Spirit* of it all. Hal Borland said, "All walking is discovery." Olympic runner Dave Bedford talked about getting out on his run and "just moving smoothly in the sunlight." Sue Browder added, "Biking invigorates and brings you in touch with what's happening around you and in tune with nature."

Still others have expressed the spirit of active living in their own special ways. The Russian poet Yevgeny Yevtushenko talked of rock climbing, a sport that offers great exhilaration to match its fierce demands. "I like the feel of the rope binding me to my comrades somewhere near the clouds," he wrote. "I like to feel the sensation of conquering the sky, although, in the final analysis, it always wins the victory over us."

Then there's Juha Vaatainen, a Finnish distance runner, who said, "I don't like to go around a track. Outside of competition I never do it. Actually stadiums were built for spectators, not for runners. We have nature and that's much better."

This connection to nature is a recurring theme—it's the *Sense of place* I alluded to. While physical activity in the gym or on the court can be invigorating and challenging, activity in a natural environment brings with it some very special feelings.

Take rowing, for example. When you're out on the water in your scull, nature is all around you—the soaring eagles, the trees along the shore, and the swamps with their bullrushes, lily pads, and unseen but teeming life. As you row along, you don't so much observe the seasons as participate in them. There is the continual reminder that we humans are not the masters of the world. We are part of it. Although there is no guarantee of a carryover effect—that a greater appreciation of nature will lead to more respect for it—I believe it increases the odds.

Bill McKibben wrote eloquently of this in *The Age of Missing Information*. To research his book, he carried out a not-so-simple experiment. With the help of the taping capabilities of a cable television network, he compared the information received (and what he learned) from watching 24 hours of television on 93 channels with what he captured in 24 hours spent on and around Crow Mountain in the Adirondacks, in upstate New York.

On the outdoor side of it, he wrote,

We can't go live in the woods by a lake—but we can go there long enough to listen, to hear. And come back not chastened but uplifted. So that we bike to work not because we have to but because it's the richest alternative. So that we live with less not because an economy in recession forces us to compromise but out of a distaste for the insulation from the real that "too much" ensures. That we grow some of our food not because we couldn't buy it but for the meeting with nature it affords and the sweetness of corn fresh picked. The question is not "Did the Indians have it right?" The question is not "Did the Amish have it right?" The question is "Can we, blessed with technology but also with nature, get it right?"

This getting it right is the *Simplicity* part. Active living affords us many choices. We *can* choose activities that require less equipment, rather than more. Activities that cost less—or nothing at all. Activities that are simple, gentle, and caring of the world around us.

By extension, the pursuit of simple, *meaningful* activities can lead to other realizations. Some people discover they no longer need to have so many things when they can derive so much happiness and satisfaction from something they do. And whether they know it or not, people who feel (and act) this way are part of the trend toward voluntary simplicity—a desire for fewer things, but more time; a less-filled but fuller life.

Active living is part of this fuller life. What you choose to do for it is entirely up to you. If you're just getting started, just getting into active living, it may be hard to imagine where it's all leading. Up to the corner and back without getting out of breath may be the first step toward some physical activity experiences, accomplishments, even adventures you never dreamed possible.

GUIDE TO QUALITY FITNESS APPRAISALS AND PHYSICAL ACTIVITY ADVICE

In Australia

Look for individuals registered with the Australian Association for Exercise and Sports Science (AAESS). AAESS registers graduates from recognized tertiary programs in exercise and sports science. For more information, you may contact AAESS, c/o Department of Biomedical Sciences, University of Wollongong, Northfields Avenue, Wollongong NSW 2522; telephone (042) 213881; fax (042) 214096.

In Canada

Look for individuals registered with the National Fitness Appraisal Certification and Accreditation (FACA) Program. The program trains individuals as either Standardized Test of Fitness Appraisers (STFA) or Certified Fitness Appraisers (CFA). Through the FACA program, facilities demonstrating high standards can also apply for status as Accredited Fitness Appraisal Centres (AFAC). For more information on individuals and facilities registered in your area, contact the Canadian Society for Exercise Physiology, 1600 James Naismith Dr., Suite 311, Gloucester, ON K1B 5N4; telephone (613) 748-5768; fax (613) 748-5763.

In New Zealand
Contact your Regional Sports Trust for information on individuals and organizations in your area offering fitness appraisals and advice.

In the United Kingdom
The British Association of Sport and Exercise Sciences (BASES) holds a register of individuals with expertise in exercise testing and fitness program design. For details, contact BASES, 114 Cardigan Road, Headingley, Leeds LS6 3BJ; telephone 0532 307558; fax 0532 755019. S/NVQs (which are being used in the UK to assure quality services across a wide range of industries) are being piloted in exercise and fitness. Wherever possible, you should use an instructor who has obtained a S/NVQ level II in teaching and instructing.

In the United States
Look for individuals certified by the American College of Sports Medicine (ACSM). The ACSM certifies individuals involved in health and fitness exercise programs and in cardiovascular rehabilitative exercise programs. Certifications include the ACSM Exercise Specialist™ and the ACSM Exercise Test Technologist™. The ACSM will also soon have in place an accreditation program for health/fitness facilities. For more information, you may contact the ACSM at Box 1440, Indianapolis, Indiana 46206-1440; telephone (317) 637-9200; fax (317) 634-7817.

SUGGESTED READING

The sampling of books here, available from your local bookstore, covers a range of topics under the active living/health umbrella. Some books are classics in their fields or long-time favorites that are regularly revised. Others are relative newcomers, offering fresh and useful information in a growing field or breaking new ground.

For advice on other reputable books, talk to a fitness specialist or other health professional. When assessing the merits of any book, always consider the qualifications and experience of the author as well as the suitability of the information to your own needs and interests.

EXERCISE AND FITNESS

These titles take a structured approach to traditional exercise programs.

The Aerobics Way by Kenneth H. Cooper (published by Bantam) is one in a series of books by Dr. Cooper that helped spark the fitness revolution.

Current popular titles from Human Kinetics include the *ACSM Fitness Book* prepared by the American College of Sports Medicine and *The Exercise Habit* by James Gavin.

STRENGTH, SUPPLENESS, BACK CARE, HOME EXERCISE

Stretching by Bob Anderson (published by Shelter Publications) is distributed by Random House. Human Kinetics offers *Weight Training: Steps to Success.*

Helpful back care books include Imrie and Barbuto's *The Back Power Program* (Stoddart) and the *YMCA Healthy Back Book* by the YMCA of the USA with Patricia Sammann (Human Kinetics).

AEROBIC ACTIVITIES, SPORTS, AND GAMES

This is a broad and deep field, but here are a few books for starters.

Runners and riders could look for *Fitness Running* or *Fitness Cycling* from Human Kinetics. *Anybody's Bike Book* by Tom Cuthbertson (Ten Speed Press), newly revised and updated, has been going strong since 1974!

For walking and hiking, look for Colin Fletcher's classic *The Complete Walker III* (Knopf), Harvey Manning's *Backpacking: One Step at a Time* (Vintage Books), and *The National Outdoor Leadership School Wilderness Guide. The Cross-Country Ski Book* by John Caldwell (Viking/Penguin) is a winter sport classic.

Human Kinetics' Outdoor Pursuits Series includes *Mountain Biking* and *Canoeing.* Its *In-Line Skating* book aims to teach "the skills for fun and fitness on wheels." Titles in its Steps to Success series include *Golf, Racquetball, Volleyball,* and *Swimming.*

GENERAL HEALTH, ENVIRONMENTAL AWARENESS

This is a rich field as well. The following titles demonstrate the range of books dealing with personal health:

Healthy Pleasures by Robert Ornstein and David Sobel (Addison-Wesley) explores the crucial role of pleasure in our health.

Personal Best (Rodale Press) collects for all time a variety of the wonderful columns written by the late George Sheehan, cardiologist, runner, and writer.

The Wellness Encyclopedia from the editors of the University of California, Berkeley Wellness Letter (Houghton Mifflin) provides straightforward answers for all your health and wellness questions.

Our relationship to the environment is eloquently covered in *The Age of Missing Information* by Bill McKibben (Plume/Penguin) and *Shadows in the Sun* by Wade Davis (Lone Pine Publishing).

RESEARCH REPORTS

I refer readers wishing details on the research that supports the health benefits of physical activity described throughout this book to *Toward Active Living* and *Physical Activity, Fitness, and Health*. Both titles can be obtained directly from Human Kinetics.

ACKNOWLEDGMENTS

A sincere thanks to . . .

. . . *exercise scientists and health epidemiologists.* Through their careful and continuing work, researchers who explore the frontiers of physical activity have confirmed the value of moderate-intensity activity and provided the scientific basis for the *active living* approach.

. . . *Health Canada.* I have enjoyed a long professional association with a number of the department's fitness/active living consultants, working on a wide range of projects with them. It was professionals there who coined the term *active living*, spearheaded the development of the concept, and have been instrumental in spreading its wonderful message.

. . . *the Canadian Fitness and Lifestyle Research Institute.* I have prepared a variety of educational materials for the Institute over the years. In particular, I had a three-year stint writing two series of monthly articles: *The Research File*, aimed at working professionals, and *Lifestyle Tips*, reaching the general public via community newspapers. The Institute graciously allowed me to adapt and draw on these materials in preparing this book.

...*The Alliance for Health and Fitness*. I worked with several alliance members to prepare a short booklet on *Active Living* when the concept was in its infancy. I truly profited from this sharing of ideas. Many of the seeds planted at that time have grown and become a part of this book.

. . . *ParticipACTION.* Always an advocate for active living, ParticipACTION has been encouraging people to "walk a block" for more than twenty years. My own approach to writing about physical activity and health has been influenced by my involvement in a number of resources developed by ParticipACTION.

. . . *other colleagues and friends.* Several people reviewed sections of the book (or the entire manuscript) and made valuable comments and suggestions.

Finally, I want to thank *Human Kinetics* for encouraging me to take on this project *and* for allowing me to tell it the way I wanted.

INDEX